The H.A.M.R. Manual

To Keith Fail -

Keith, I know you are going to
like this and be good at it. Let me
Know what you think.

David N___

The H.A.M.R. Manual
How to Rewire Your Own Brain

David K. Nelms

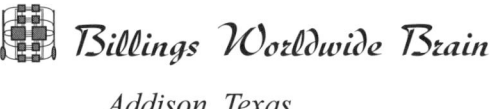 Billings Worldwide Brain

Addison, Texas

Published by

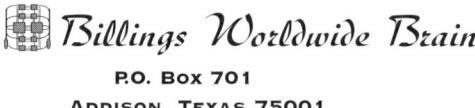

Billings Worldwide Brain

P.O. BOX 701

ADDISON, TEXAS 75001

Library of Congress Cataloging-in-Publication Data

Nelms, David K.
    The h.a.m.r. manual: how to rewire your own brain.
    Includes bibliographical references and index.
    ISBN 0-9654169-6-8 : $19.95
    1. Applied Psychology-Self Actualization.   I. Title.
    2. Attitude Change.
    3. Psychotherapy.
    4. Success.
BF637.S4.N423 1997   158.1   96-86026

Printed in the United States of America
10 9 8 7 6 5 4 3 2 1

Acknowledgment

Many people have contributed to the formation of this book in some way or another, and their efforts are sincerely appreciated. It is impossible to mention all of them, but a few of those who bear recognition are as follows: C.D. Nelms, MD; John Monturo, EdD, LPC, NCC; Jane Conway; R.J. Nelms, MD; Lance Baker MBE; W.E. Litle DDS; Patty Evans; Glenda Raver; Steve Dunavant.

To my beloved Jane

Warning

This book describes a process that has been shown to have powerful effects on the human brain. Neither the publisher nor the author are engaged in rendering psychiatric advice or medical services. If psychiatric or medical services or advice are needed, you should seek out qualified licensed professional care.

Due to the newness of the system there have been no long term studies to quantify its effects. Every effort is made to convey the information necessary to use HAMR as safely as possible; however, there may be mistakes both typographical and in content. Any use of this system is at your own risk.

No responsibility can be assumed by the author or the publisher for the use or misuse of the information contained in this book. David Nelms and Billings Worldwide Brain shall have no liability or responsibility to any person or legal entity with respect to any loss or damage incurred from reading or using this manual.

If you do not understand the warning, or do not wish to be bound to the above, this book may be returned to Billings Worldwide Brain for a full and instantaneous refund. This book may be returned at any time for any reason.

Contents

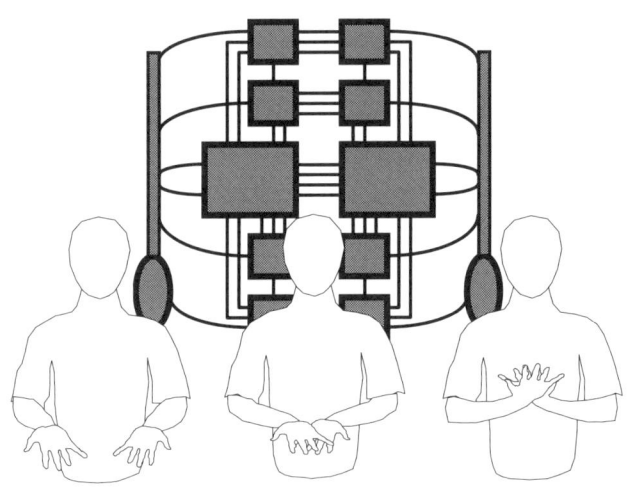

Four rules for the aspiring author of a scientific article:
#1 Have something to say
#2 Say it
#3 Stop as soon as you have said it
#4 Give the paper a proper title
Dr. John Shaw Billings, founder of National Library of Medicine and Index Medicus

Hand Actuated Mental Reconditioning (HAMR)

Many people are constantly striving to improve themselves in some way or another. They learn all they can from self-help books and sink thousands of dollars into seminars, tapes and personal trainers or therapists. Some of these things work well for people, and their practitioners are genuinely dedicated to helping others, but too often the result is frustration and wasted time and money. For the practitioner of psychotherapy who strives to help others, there is also frustration in that most systems are only marginally effective and require prohibitive amounts of time and effort to accomplish. What is needed is a system for reprogramming the human mind that is fast, easy and is based on the wiring of the brain. This book provides such a system, in a format that is simple to learn and understand.

Illustrations depict the system by briefly describing the brain, HAMR theory, the steps and a few recommendations on getting started on various situations. The HAMR Manual is something of a picture book in that the *text serves only to fill in details for the illustrations*. It is strongly recommended that you **go through and carefully study all of the pictures and their captions before reading the text-portion.**

Rewiring your own brain is easy if you know how, and learning how is easy with this book. Take your time and go over the diagrams as many times as you need to in order to thoroughly grasp the system. Learn it inside and out, and there will be no limit to what you can accomplish for your brain. You will understand how to apply HAMR to any situation that may arise. Having the ability to rewire your own brain will give you an edge, and it will quickly become your most precious and indispensable commodity.

This book will stimulate the interest of research-minded individuals and brain theorists as well as people who just want to improve themselves. HAMR is a system that can be neatly quantified and tested under controlled conditions. The steps are applied in the same manner for every person all of the time, and the results are astounding. The implications of this phenomena are far reaching.

Having the ability to rewire your own brain will put you in much firmer control of your destiny. By giving your brain good, positive programs to work with, you will enable it to demonstrate that its potential is virtually unlimited. Get ready for a whole new ball game.

2

The Brain

The theory behind the HAMR system is based on neurology. It was derived from a study of the most current scientific models of the brain. Therefore, a brief summary of how the brain is thought to work is in order. This chapter is not intended to be an Atlas to Neurology. It is intended only to provide an understanding of the brain that strikes a balance somewhere between accuracy, simplicity and HAMR theory.

The more you understand about how the brain works, the better you are able to make HAMR perform. Studying other sources on the subject of neurology is highly recommended. Left Brain Right Brain, by Springer and Deutsch is a very good book that is easy to understand and comprehensive in its scope.

Overview. The first thing you might notice if you looked at a brain are the **cerebral hemispheres**. They are the big, gray lumpy parts that are most visible. The cerebral hemispheres are also called the neocortex. Higher faculties such as abstract reasoning and language originate here. The neocortex is comprised of two cerebral hemispheres that are essentially mirror images of each other (in a gross anatomical sense).

Reptiles do not have any developed neocortex, except for the Nile crocodile, which has a tiny one. Birds have small ones, and can do amazing things with them. The largest and most complex cerebral hemispheres, however, belong to the mammals. The biggest ones are in dolphins and killer whales, followed closely by humans. The rest of the primates trail a bit farther behind.

The HAMR Diagram. To facilitate the imagination we bring you the HAMR Diagram. It serves to provide a means of visualizing the human brain at work. The cerebral hemispheres are divided into lobes that carry out somewhat discreet functions. Each lobe is represented by its own picture screen. The screens are wired together in a way that is similar to the actual connections in the brain. It is not exact by any means, but it will convey a general idea of how the lobes are connected together.

The squares in the diagram represent vast organizations of neurons in the "skin" of the cerebral cortex. These organizations of neurons are in huge, flat sheets. Each sheet of neurons has about five layers. The layers perform differing functions, which consist mainly of communicating with other neurons at various distances. Some layers have connections to neurons very close, and some connect to other areas of the brain altogether.

HAMRscreens

The HAMR diagrams are based on the premise that columns in the neocortex can be compared to the pixels on a TV screen.

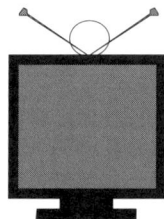

Pictures on the screens represent patterns on the neocortex and hippocampus.

Neurons across the surface of the brain are also organized into columns. The columns operate as groups, and they are standing side by side, packed together tightly. For the purposes of this book, we compare these columns to pixels on a TV screen. If you get close to a television the pixels are visible as small dots or squares. The diagram is devised with this metaphor in mind.

Like pixels on a TV screen, the activities of single columns mean something only when taken in the context of other columns. When you look very closely at a TV screen you can see individual pixels flashing colors. From a greater distance the colors become a picture. The surface of the brain uses a similar technique with its columns. Patterns emerge from the uproar of chaotically firing columns in the same way that moving images form from the coordinated flashing of television pixels.

The surface of the brain, or cerebral hemispheres, is much

Diagram of HAMR

The Diagram of HAMR is a simplified schematic of the neocortex and some of its largest connections. It is used as an aid in describing the theoretical objectives of HAMR.

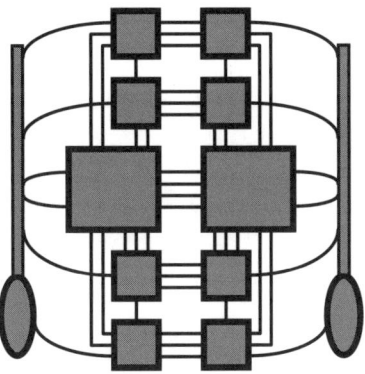

The scenarios shown on the screens are not an accurate depiction of neurological activity; they were devised to simplify an almost hopelessly complicated subject.

more complex than a single TV screen. A thousand screens that are capable of communicating with each other would be closer to the mark. Our simplified schematic model of the hemispheres will shamelessly reduce it to twelve.

From the top screen and working downward, we have the occipital lobe, the parietal lobe, the huge frontal lobe, the cingulate gyrus, and the temporal lobe. Each of these areas consists of a right side and a left side that are wired completely together. The spoon-shaped images on the sides represent the hippocampi.

Cortex. The term *gray matter* refers to the "skin" (or outer layer) of the hemispheres. If you were to peel off this skin and squash it flat it would be about the size of a checkerboard. It consists of about nine billion neurons that are organized into layers and columns.

The layers consist of neurons that have different functions. These functions largely pertain to sending fibers to other parts of the brain and spinal cord. Some layers have neurons that communicate with others that are close to them, and some have

---

Chaos on Screen

The squares in the HAMR diagram represent the lobes of the brain, as if you could lay them flat and observe simplified versions of their activity.

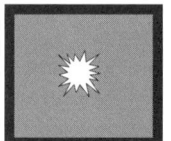 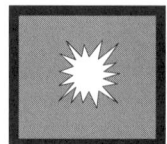 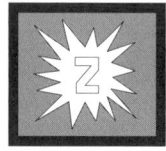 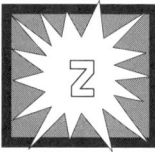

Elevated activity is represented by starbursts of varying sizes.
The **leftmost** screen is at rest,
the **second** screen has become excited,
the **third** screen depicts a pattern of activity **(Z)**,
the **rightmost** screen shows such a high level of activity that accelerated learning occurs, and the strength of the pattern is increased.

neurons that stretch to other areas, near and far. The longest stretch of any is from the motor strip all the way down to the base of the spine.

Areas on one side of the cerebral cortex are wired directly to equivalent areas on the other. The bundle of fibers that accomplishes this task is called the corpus callosum.

The cerebral hemispheres are divided into lobes, and each one has a different set of functions. Some lobes receive input directly from sensory organs like ears, eyes, nose, skin and visceral organs. Others have "motor" areas and provide the signals that instruct muscles to flex. Some parts of these lobes combine and integrate the signals from several other areas at once. These are called association areas.

Occipital Lobes. The primary visual area is at the occipital pole, located at the very back of the brain. The eyes connect to this area, and each side of it receives half of the picture. In other words if you focus your eyes in a given direction, everything you see in the left half of the picture is being processed by your right occipital lobe, and everything you see on the right is processed by your left occipital lobe.

The image you see with your eyes is comprised of the cooperative efforts of the columns that reside in the primary visual

---

Areas of Cortex Stimulate Each Other

Connected areas of cortex stimulate each other. HAMR uses this phenomenon to raise activity levels high enough to strengthen new and more desirable patterns.

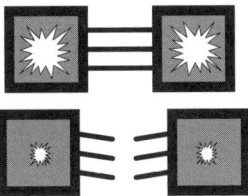

If an area is isolated from all other areas, it will become quiet and inactive (bottom).

cortex. The occipital lobes are directly wired to the frontal lobes, which also play a key part in sight and the visualization of ideas.

Parietal Lobes. The primary kinesthetic sensory area is the parietal lobe's foremost claim to fame. The entire body is mapped on the parietal lobes several times. Everything you feel

---

Facilitation and Inhibition

Neurons and groups of neurons communicate through sending and receiving chemicals called neurotransmitters. When a cell receives a little packet of these chemicals, it can be affected in one of two possible ways:

> **A** it becomes more active (facilitation), or
> **B** it becomes less active (inhibition).

Large groups of cells use a combination of these two effects and form complex patterns with them. Some neurological pathways lean more towards one effect than the other. A way to think of it is that facilitation communicates by beaming light, and inhibition communicates by casting shadow. The net result can be highly detailed patterns of light and dark, like a black and white photograph.

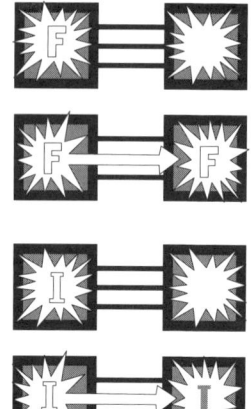

Facilitation (F) is shown as light patterns being transmitted to another square,

Inhibition (I) is depicted as dark patterns being transmitted to another square.

Electrical pulses are generated and conducted by neurons, but meaningful neurological communications between cells depend on facilitation and inhibition.

with your skin and muscles is being processed in these lobes first. They are also involved with logical operations such as math and language comprehension, and a good part of their real estate is taken up with associating signals from other areas.

Temporal Lobes. The temporal lobes are the center of hearing where the primary auditory areas are located. Speech, musical ability, and concepts of time are a few of the processes that take place here. As with every process in the brain, the responsibility is shared by other areas also.

Each ear is connected to the temporal lobe on the other side of the brain from it, with some fibers also stopping on the same side. The temporal lobes are suspected to be heavily involved with emotion and memory as well.

Occipital Lobes

The top screens represent the occipital lobes, which are located at the posterior end of the brain (toward the back of the head). The occipital lobes receive input directly from the eyes. Raw visual information(V) is processed into more usable forms and passed along to many other areas of the brain.

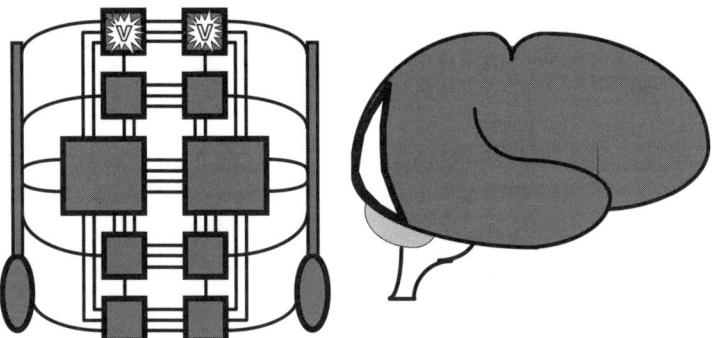

The eyes are connected directly to the primary visual cortex, which is located at the occipital pole. Each eye is divided into two halves, and each half is connected to the opposite side of the brain, so that everything you see to the left of center is coming from the right side of your brain, and everything you see to the right of center is coming from the left side of your brain.

Cingulate Gyrus. The cingulate gyrus is not considered a "lobe," but the Diagram of HAMR makes it look that way. It is located on the inside surfaces of the hemispheres. You have to split the brain in half to see them. They arch over the corpus callosum, and they are associated with various aspects of the emotional processes.

Frontal Lobes. The frontal lobes are the largest of all lobes in humans. They are huge in relation to the rest of the brain. In addition to being big, they have large bundles of fibers that connect them directly to all of the other lobes. The frontal lobes are associated with future planning, motor activity, emotional responses, and visualization.

The motor strip is located along the edge that runs into the parietal lobe. It provides the signals that directly inspire muscles to contract. The signals it sends are modulated by an area called the cerebellum. The cerebellum is not shown in the Diagram of HAMR.

Parietal Lobes

The second set of screens represents the parietal lobes. The sensory strips at the anterior edge of these lobes process and distribute tactile or kinesthetic information **(K)** that they receive from nerves in the skin and muscles of the body.

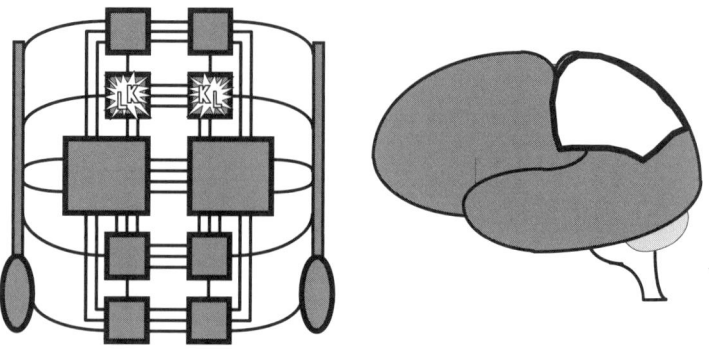

The parietal lobes also contribute logical operations **(L)** such as math and are involved with the comprehension of speech.

Hippocampus. Memory is a complicated issue, but the hippocampus is involved with both long term and short term storage. More than likely it stores a skeletal or compressed version of a memory, and the cerebral cortex stores and fills in the details. The hippocampus consists of two separate structures that are each located on a different side of the brain. Each one is buried deep in the temporal lobe and is connected to many areas of the cortex.

Corpus Callosum. The bundle of fibers that connects the hemispheres together most directly is called the corpus callosum. It is the largest bundle of fibers in the brain. On the dia-

Frontal Lobes

The center set of screens represents the frontal lobes. Note that they are robustly wired to the other areas. The motor strip at the posterior edge of this lobe enervates the skeletal muscles of the body.

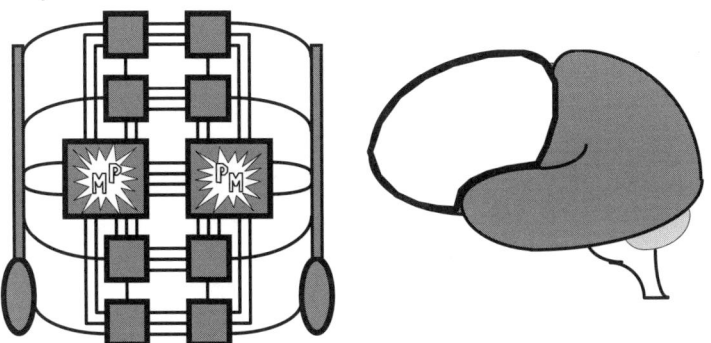

The frontal lobes are also involved in memory, emotion, and concepts having to do with "the future". Broca's area, which is involved with generating language, is located there as well.

The two sides are also specialized for different types of functioning, such as holistic versus detail-oriented thinking, and approach versus withdrawal aspects of planning.

In addition to planning(**P**) and motor function(**M**), the frontal lobes contain areas that associate information from other parts of the brain. For this reason they are a central fixture of HAMR.

gram it is the row of wires that runs down the middle. The callosum allows the two sides of the brain to communicate directly to each other, although without it much information still manages to pass from side to side.

The callosum is thought to allow the hemispheres to communicate through inhibition. In some cases it may be used to integrate information together, such as details and the big picture, but more often it probably allows the each side to reduce the activity of the other. When both hemispheres are of equal strength they should be able to balance each other out in this

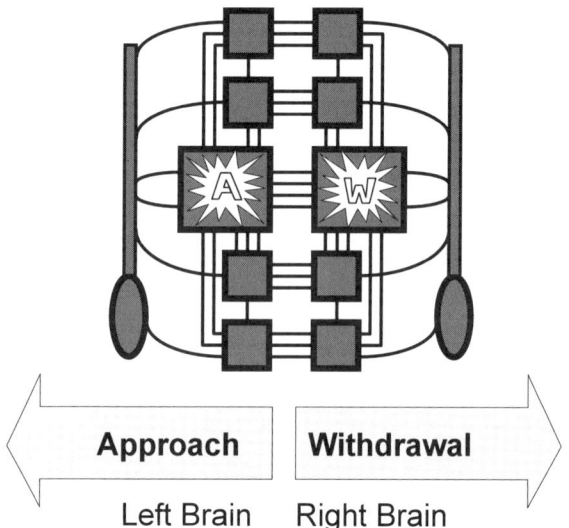

Approach~Withdrawal and the Brain

The anterior frontal lobes are thought to be specialized for approach versus withdrawal behaviors.

Approach   **Withdrawal**

Left Brain   Right Brain

Joy Interest Desire Anger   **Terror Fear Distress Disgust**

The effects of approach-computations are experienced more to the right side of the body, and the effects of withdrawal-computations are experienced more to the left side of the body.

manner.

Some forms of severe epilepsy have been treated by severing the callosum surgically. This has afforded brain researchers the opportunity to gain valuable information regarding its role. Amazingly, the effects of cutting the corpus callosum are nearly undetectable to the untrained eye. A person can evidently do very well without it. Early brain researchers were even prompted to joke that "the only purpose of the corpus callosum is to keep the two sides of the brain from falling apart."

Older Structures. If you were to slice a brain right down the middle you would get a be able to view some of the other major parts of the brain. Most easily recognizable are some structures known as the **hindbrain and midbrain**. These are the oldest part of the brain. They are either responsible for or greatly involved with unconscious or automatic aspects of behavior. Breathing, sleep cycles, heart rate, and general degree of arousal

---

The Approach~Withdrawal Continuum

Darwin suggested that all behaviors be divided into two functional groups: approach and withdrawal.

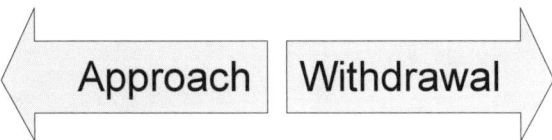

Joy Interest Desire Anger / Terror Fear Distress Disgust

In the event of "withdrawal" type behavior an organism retracts from the environment or freezes. Fear, disgust and distress are emotions that are used to facilitate withdrawal type behavior.

In the event of "approach" type behavior an organism moves to engage the environment. Some emotions which facilitate approach strategies are anger, joy, and interest.

All complex interactions with the environment are produced by some mixture of these two operations.

are some examples.

Chaos. Areas of cerebral cortex are connected together in precise ways. Any two areas that are united by large bundles of fibers will stimulate each other to activity. This activity is chaotic in nature. The squares of the diagram represent given areas of cerebral cortex that are connected directly together. Under normal circumstances these areas stimulate and feed each others' activity.

An article by Walter J. Freeman[1] discusses the action of chaos in the brain and describes some experiments that illustrate the point:

In one experiment two cell groups are disconnected from each other by severing the fibers between them. Both groups became quiet and inactive, suggesting that groups of neurons communicate with each other but they also need each other to re-

Cingulate Gyrus

The cingulate gyrus is located in the split between the brain-halves. It works closely with a number of older areas in producing emotion.

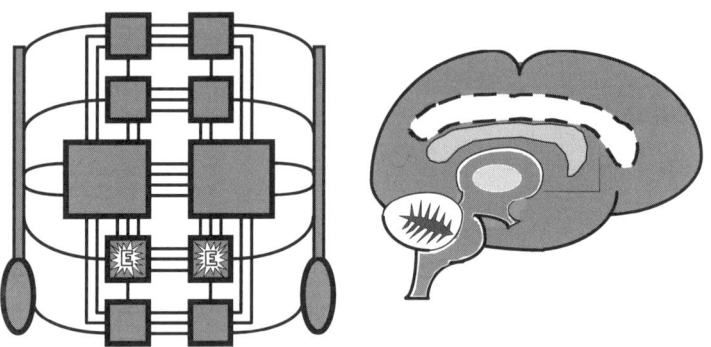

The cingulate gyrus is not considered to be a lobe, but for purposes of HAMR it is given its own set of screens. We think of the left gyrus as moderating approach related emotions like anger, interest and desire, and the right gyrus as moderating withdrawal emotions such as fear, distress, and disgust.

main stimulated.

In another experiment a grid of electrodes was arrayed over the olfactory bulb of a rabbit. The rabbit was exposed to various different smells. Patterns of activity were contour mapped to reveal the "shapes" of the chaotic bursts that resulted. After establishing which smell produced what shape, the rabbit was subjected to training.

First the rabbit was trained to associate the smell of sawdust with a certain stimulus. Next the animal was taught to recognize the smell of a banana. Lastly, the rabbit was exposed to the smell of sawdust once again, but this time the mapped pattern of bulbar activity had changed, altered by learning in the rest of the brain.

Freeman therefore concludes that the activity of the olfactory bulb is dominated more by experience than by stimuli. Possibly the experience of many parts of the brain combine to produce this effect. Learning by the brain affects the shapes of

Temporal Lobes

The bottom screens represent the temporal lobes which receive input from the ears. In addition to hearing, they process concepts of time, music, and are involved with the comprehension of speech.

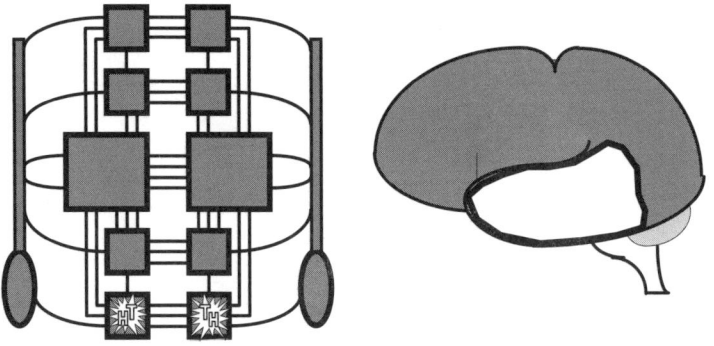

In addition to hearing(**H**), concepts of time and tempo(**T**) are processed here.

patterns at the olfactory bulb, all the way out in the nose of the rabbit.

In other words, when a given area of the brain is connected to another given area, the activity of each area will affect the activity of the other. If one hundred brain areas are connected, the aggregate pattern of activity would reflect the presence and mood of all one hundred at the same time.

A very few neurons firing in a particular pattern can send millions, if not billions of neurons into firing with a larger pattern. A few smell molecules can send your whole brain into an instant explosion of alarm if those molecules belong to smoke coming out of your kitchen.

Consider the humble rabbit, or any mammal for that matter. It has a nose with olfactory receptor-type neurons and an olfactory bulb positioned above said receptor neurons. The bulb has an olfactory tract that connects it to the rest of the brain.

Hippocampus

The hippocampus is buried deep inside the temporal lobe and is involved in long and short term memory**(P)**.

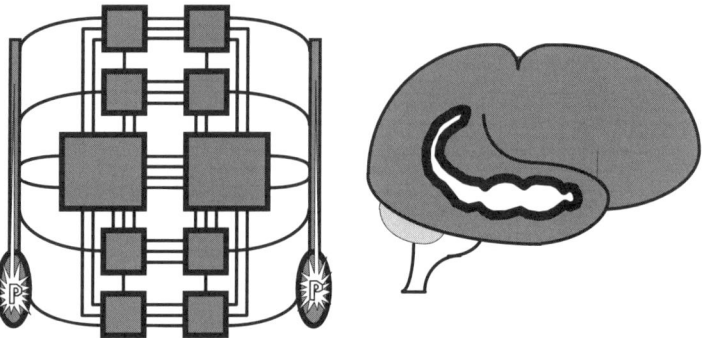

It is connected to areas all over the brain but has its strongest associations with the temporal lobes, frontal lobes and cingulate gyrus. It is likely that a skeletal representation of memory is retained by the hippocampus, and that details such as sights, sounds, and feelings are retained in newer structures of the neocortex (as described in previous diagrams).

What you might think is that a certain smell, let's say sawdust, would trigger the receptor neuron to send the bulb a signal that means "sawdust". Then the bulb would get a pattern that means "sawdust" and send that to the brain.

However, it does not work that way. Even at this first identification of smell, the entire brain has instantly participated in analyzing and identifying the odor. The pattern of activity at the olfactory bulb reflects the activity of the whole brain.

Here is an example that you can demonstrate to yourself: hold a pencil in your mouth sideways like a bit would be fitted in a horse's mouth, and bite down for a few seconds. The muscles in your jaw and face contract in a way that is similar to the contractions necessary for a smile. The result is a slight feeling of happiness or well being.

Corpus Callosum

The corpus callosum is a massive bundle of nerve fibers that connects the cerebral hemispheres directly together.

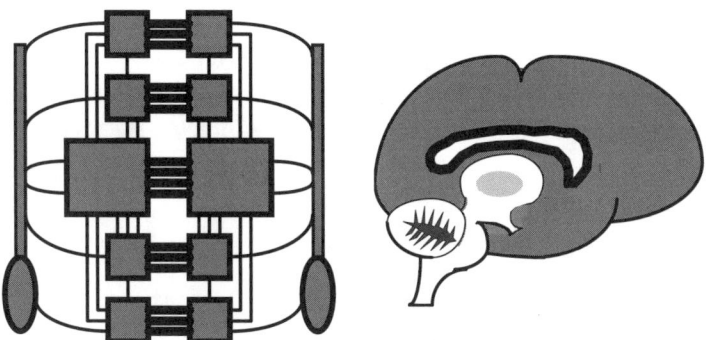

When performing a task, each side of the brain processes different aspects of information. Through the callosum, each side of the brain remains constantly aware of the activities of the other. The two hemispheres can therefore work in unison, and there is a division of labor.

The callosum is thought to work largely through inhibition. Each hemisphere "casts a shadow" of its activity through the corpus callosum.

In another example, if you hold a pencil in your mouth with pursed lips (as if holding a cigar), some of the muscles involved with frowning are activated. The resulting cerebral action elicits feelings associated with frowning. A very few neurons are sensing a tiny fraction of "smile" or "frown" patterns, and as a result the whole brain participates.

The point to all this is actually rather simple. The brain is huge and complicated, with many functional areas, but they all work together as a whole unit. Learning is accomplished by new patterns being established across the entire brain at once. Any therapy or mental reprogramming method will have to take this phenomena into account.

If you try to install a new pattern into only a small portion of the brain at once, it will not have the opportunity to become permanent. A small and insecure pattern will be overwhelmed by a larger and more well established pattern every time. This is why "willpower" is no match for establishing permanent change in the personality. The HAMR system is designed to

The Brain Stem

The oldest areas of the brain are a large collection of nerve pathways and nuclei called the brain stem. It is comprised of many important structures but is largely ignored in this book.

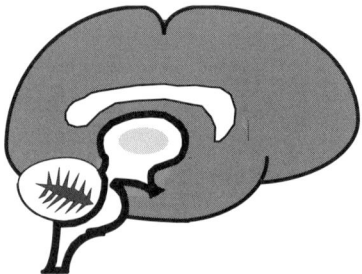

The brain stem is not represented in the Diagram of HAMR because it is not directly targeted by HAMR. This does not diminish its role by any means, however, for it actually remains a vital contributor in all operations.

install patterns across the entire cerebral cortex at once.

Synapses. Neurons communicate with each other through little connectors called synapses. They are located at the ends of the branches that extend from neuron to neuron. Electricity in the form of pulses travels from the body of a cell out to the ends of the branches (called axons). When a pulse gets to the end of a branch, a little packet of chemicals shoots across to the other cell.

The packet contains chemicals called neurotransmitters. Neurotransmitters cause the next neuron in the line to generate a burst which in turn travels to that neurons body. In this way electricity travels all over the brain and accomplishes amazing things.

Some synapses connect neurons from area to area, and others connect cells next to each other. Synapses connecting neurons

The Hemispheres are Specialized for Different Aspects of a Given Task

The two sides of the brain combine forces to achieve a given mission. The right brain deals with "the big picture", and the left brain deals with more "detail oriented" information.

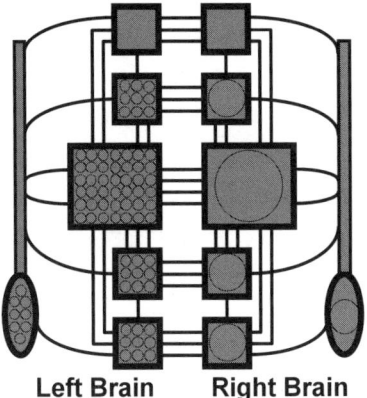

Left Brain   Right Brain

An example is speech; wherein the left brain deals with wording and syntax, and the right brain deals with tonal quality and emotional content.

within groups are the mediators of patterns, and are called Hebbian synapses. Hebbian synapses are the connectors between cells that sculpt electricity into meaningful shapes.

Cells that are connected to each other can influence each other in two ways: facilitation and inhibition. In the case of facilitation one cell encourages the other to be active. In the case of inhibition one cell stops the other from firing. Both effects are necessary to produce electrical shapes on the neocortex and in deeper parts of the brain.

Consider the way shadows and light areas combine to make pictures on a black and white TV screen. The light areas are experiencing more facilitation, and the shadowed areas are experiencing more inhibition. Together they make pictures that we can see and comprehend.

Approach-Withdrawal. Charles Darwin[2] was one of the first to suggest that behavior can be considered in terms of two in-

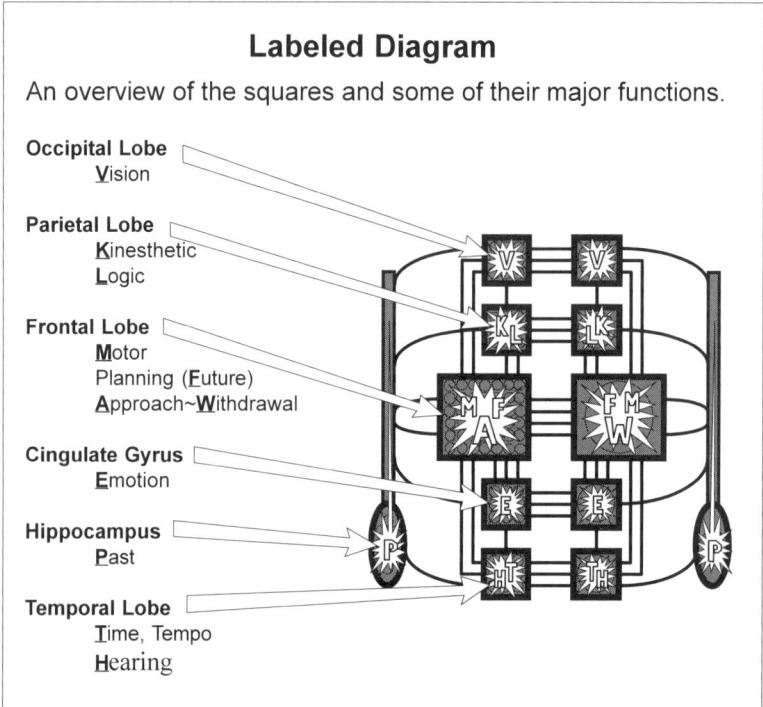

Labeled Diagram

An overview of the squares and some of their major functions.

Occipital Lobe
    Vision

Parietal Lobe
    Kinesthetic
    Logic

Frontal Lobe
    Motor
    Planning (Future)
    Approach~Withdrawal

Cingulate Gyrus
    Emotion

Hippocampus
    Past

Temporal Lobe
    Time, Tempo
    Hearing

teracting strategies: approach and withdrawal. All of the emotions can be divided by function into one of these two groups. Every interaction with the environment consists of a delicate dance between the two.

Feelings like anger, interest, and joy all encourage interaction with the environment. They are classified as approach related emotions. Anger is the most powerful, as it results in a more robust approach. Interest brings about exploration, and joy brings about personal interaction.

At the other end of the scale are the emotions that foster withdrawal from the environment. Fear, distress, and disgust are in this category. Perhaps abject terror would be most potent. These emotions all bring about a hasty retreat or "freezing up" in many cases.

To properly capitalize on any situation, you need to have at

Communication within Hemispheres

The brain is divided down the middle into two distinct hemispheres. The circuits within the brain communicate via a mixture of facilitation and inhibition, but communication between different areas of the same hemisphere may lean more towards facili-

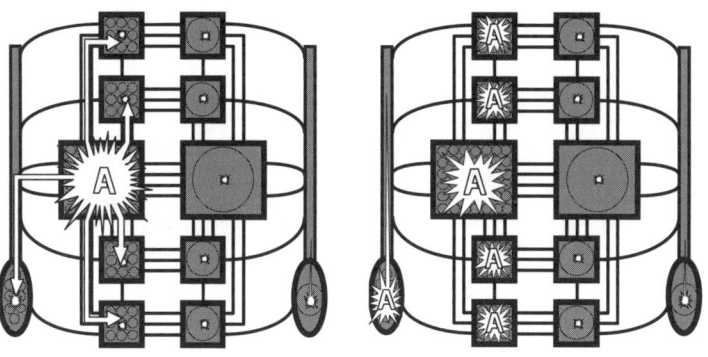

tation.

At left: the left frontal lobe becomes excited with a pattern **(A)**.
At right: the light (facilitory) pattern has been communicated to the other connected areas. The net effect of this communication is an increase in activity throughout the cortex.

your disposal the full range of emotional response. Emotions are the power-packs of the brain, and you must be able to utilize them all if you want maximum performance from your equipment.

There is strong evidence[3] to suggest that the anterior portions of the frontal lobes are specialized for approach and withdrawal functions. The left frontal lobe performs approach calculations, and the right frontal lobe performs withdrawal calculations. This configuration is apparently present at birth.

Measuring the activity a person has across the anterior frontal lobes[4] can predict general disposition or "affective style" of that person. People with relatively more activity in the left anterior frontal lobes report more approach type emotions (posi-

---

Communication between Hemispheres

The two halves of the brain are connected to each other area by area. The bundle of fibers that connect them is called the corpus collosum, and it is thought to use primarily inhibition to send its signals.

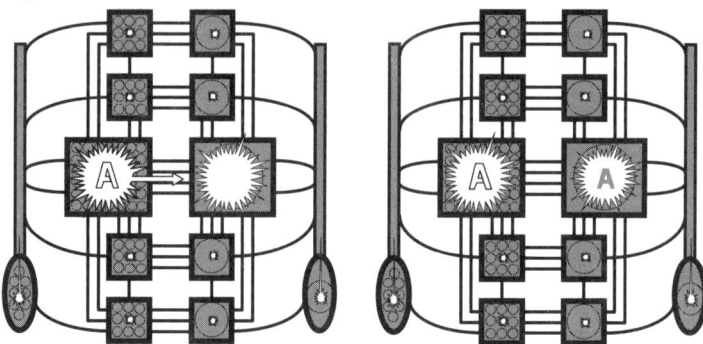

Left: the left frontal lobe is excited with pattern **(A)**.
Right: through inhibition the pattern is communicated to the frontal lobe on the other side of the brain. The net effect of this communication is a decrease in the activity of the right frontal lobe.

When both frontal lobes are performing in a sound manner, they will monitor as well as moderate each other's activity. This results in a healthy balance of operation.

tive affect), and people with relatively more activity in the right anterior frontal lobes report more withdrawal emotions (negative affect).

Studies at the University of Wisconsin-Madison[5] have turned up solid links between depression and underactivity of the left anterior lobe. Henriques and Davidson propose that this "pattern of diminished left-sided frontal activation indicates a deficit in approach mechanisms in depressed subjects." Other stud-

---

Learning

During neurological operations, the brain can use patterns that are learned (strong), or patterns that are unlearned (weak). Learned patterns are shown with heavy surrounding lines, and unlearned patterns with thin surrounding lines.

Unlearned patterns are thin and weak. They have an insubstantial number of synapses to support them, and they are unlikely to be recalled easily.

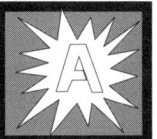

Learned patterns are chemically established in the connections between neurons, and over time new branches may grow to strengthen them further. Normally, they can be rapidly recalled to activation.

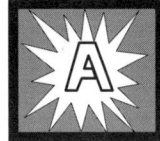

For practical purposes, strengthening of a pattern (learning), can occur as a result of any of three fundamental circumstances:

> **#1 repetitive use:** the pattern receives repeated reinforcement
> **#2 the Hebb Rule:** the pattern brings about a reward
> **#3 traumatic event:** neurological activity is brought above a certain level, and the brainstem pumps out a dose of pattern-reinforcing chemicals

Since repetitive use is not a significant part of the HAMR system, it will largely be omitted from further discussion.

ies[6] have also reached similar conclusions.

Lower self esteem is also linked to greater right hemispherisity[7] in a study at Laurentian University. According to Persinger and Makarec, "People who reported the greatest numbers of right hemispheric indicators displayed the lowest self esteem."

Recent experiments with imaging techniques strengthen the concept of the approach-withdrawal continuum. Researchers have shown that the left and right anterior frontal lobes are specialized for this setup. The left side of your brain is specialized for approach behavior, and the right side of your brain is specialized for withdrawal behavior. This applies mostly to the frontal lobes, but HAMR theory assumes that it extends also to the parietal lobes, temporal lobes, and cingulate gyrus.

It has been demonstrated that depression is associated with underactivity of the left anterior frontal lobe, and/or a deficit of approach-related behavior. Studies exist which link the suppression of anger to elevations in blood pressure, and the over-expression of anger to coronary malfunction.

In summary, the research that has been done by these fine people tells us many interesting things. The human brain is a diverse and complex electrical machine that operates as a single unit. Patterns at one end of the brain are affected by activity at the other end of the brain.

The brain can be divided down the center into halves. The two halves perform different functions. In order to have a balanced life, you must have a balanced brain. One half of the brain performs calculations that deal with advancement, and the other half of the brain performs calculations that deal with retreat. To deal effectively with life's diversity of situations, both sides of the brain are needed. To suppress the activity of a given set of emotions is to suppress the activity of one side of the brain. Though it seems like good idea at the time, the result of this practice is mental instability, insanity, and sickness.

What is needed is a way to install more useful patterns into the whole brain at once. The new patterns should utilize both halves of the brain with equal enthusiasm. In the next chapter, we will explore how that can be done.

---

[1]"The Physiology of Perception" by Walter J. Freeman MD Scientific American 1991

[2]Darwin, C.R. (1965). *The Expression of Emotions in Man and Animals.* Chicago: University of Chicago Press. (org.pub.1872)

[3]Davidson Richard J. *Emotion and Affective Style: Hemispheric Substrates.* Psychological Science (vol.3 no.1, January 1992)

[4]Fox, Nathan A. *Electroencephalograph Asymmetry and the Development of Emotion.* American Psychologist (August 1991)

[5]Henriques, Jeffery B. and Davidson, Richard J. *Left Frontal Hypoactivation in Depression.* Journal of Abnormal Psychology (Vol. 100, No. 4, 1991)

[6]Biondi, Parise, Venturi, Riccio, Brunetti, and Pancheri. *Frontal Hemisphere Lateralization and Depressive Personality Traits.* Perceptual and Motor Skills (1993, 77, 1035-1042)

[7]Persinger,M.A., and Makarec, Katherine. *Greater Right Hemispherisity is Associated with Lower Self Esteem in Adults.*
Perceptual and Motor Skills (1991, 73, 1244-1246)

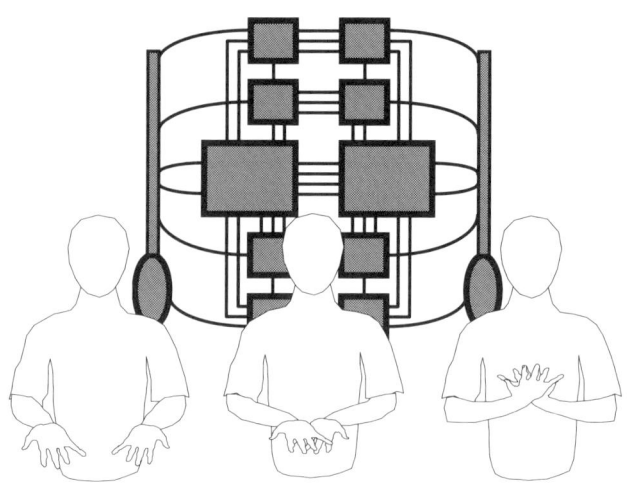

3

H.A.M.R. Theory

   The theory that drives HAMR is based on scientific principles. Some of these are somewhat new and innovative discoveries, but most are age-old tidbits of well established knowledge. The techniques were developed through analysis of the behavioral sciences and experimentation with various self-help methodologies.

   The premise of the theory is that almost all mental problems are brought about by the same psychological mechanism: one or more areas of the brain are inhibited by other areas of the brain. Most of the time the inhibited regions are in the left frontal lobe. The inhibition is brought about by learning. This learning of undesirable patterns occurs by means of either the Hebb rule or the big scare, both of which will be discussed in this chapter.

   Since the anterior frontal lobes are specialized for approach and withdrawal behaviors, it follows that determining which lobe has gone awry can be easily accomplished by examining the problem. If you have trouble asserting yourself in a given situation it is the right or withdrawal hemisphere that dominates. If you have trouble keeping your aggression in check it is the left or approach hemisphere that dominates.

Unless you are trying to outrun a swarm of killer bees, you will want to have full access to both approach and withdrawal. Thus, the best of all possible solutions is a balanced interplay between both cerebral hemispheres. This balance of hemispheric activity would be justly referred to as "finesse."

Balancing the Brain. The aim of HAMR is to create a perfectly balanced system that utilizes the entire spectrum of mental processing. No matter what you are doing, the skills necessary will be contrived of some combination of both sides of the brain. HAMR is designed to establish patterns across the cerebral cortex that make this possible.

The two hemispheres are specialized for processing different aspects of a given task. One powerful theory is that the approach-withdrawal continuum is an integral part of this spe-

---

The Hebb Rule

When a pattern of activity brings about a reward, the brain stem secretes chemicals that cause the pattern to become strengthened.

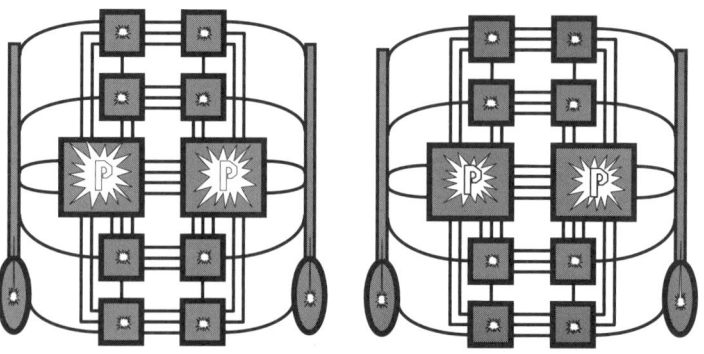

Left: the brain executes pattern **(P)**, and it works to secure a reward.
Right: chemicals from the brain stem have established pattern **(P)**, and now it is easily repeated.

cialization. An important part of this theory is that emotion "powers" these two aspects. Approach is related to anger at the one extreme, and withdrawal is related to fear at the other.

For this reason it is best to have skill in utilizing the entire range of emotion from anger to fear and everything in between. In the beginning you will set the full emotional array loose, then install the necessary software for employing it properly. Recall that your health depends on good emotional balance.

To a person that represses anger this will sound counter-intuitive and difficult to accept. But HAMR has remained hidden from mankind because it goes against human intuition. We are afraid that letting anger come out will turn us into mass murderers, yet the suppression of this emotion is what causes such problems in the first place. The brain is equipped for moderating emotional responses, but only when it functions as a whole. Integrating your anger into the activity of your entire brain will make it much more manageable.

The Will. The conscious mind is comprised of "things of which you are or can be aware." Everything *else* that goes on inside your brain, and of which you are not currently aware, is considered the "unconscious mind." The brain is large and complicated, so by far the greatest portion of activity at any given time is unconscious.

The Diagram of HAMR is thought of as representing parts of the brain that can be manipulated by the conscious mind. For purposes of HAMR the will is defined as: "conscious thought that activates a given area of cortex." By directing your thoughts to a given perception, you are activating specific areas of your brain.

Parts of the brain that are connected together are said to be *associated*. After an area of cortex has been activated, it causes other areas that are associated with it to also become activated. This action persists for a time while processing information, then eventually dies back down to a resting state.

The period of time in which activity persists is critical to the effectiveness of HAMR. The objective of the process is to excite several key areas of the brain in rapid succession. These key areas are excited one at a time by briefly concentrating on certain concepts. It only takes a thought in a given direction to activate an area of neocortex; no extended meditation is necessary or desirable.

To perform the HAMR operation a chain of specific thoughts is rapidly entertained. After one thought has been accessed momentarily, another thought in the chain is considered. This "chaining of thoughts" is executed quickly so that by the time the last area of cortex has been activated, the first area that was activated is still in a frenzy. In the end, all of the areas of the brain that have been excited are active at the same time so that they may blend their respective patterns together.

For example, when you look at something your occipital lobe fires up, when you listen to something your temporal lobe fires

Traumatic Event

When an event occurs that brings the entire brain to above a certain level of activity, the brain stem secretes chemicals that cause the pattern to become strengthened.

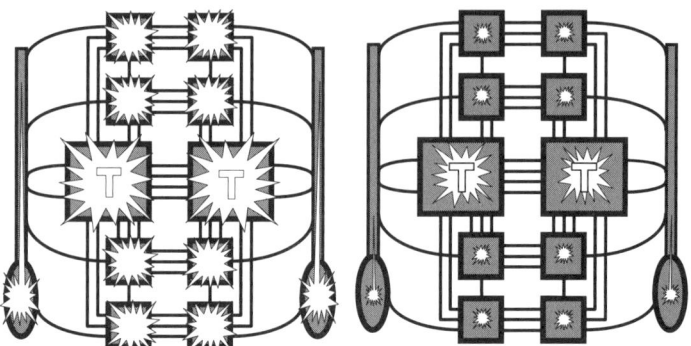

Left: pattern **(T)** is present on the neocortex during an experience that is traumatic
Right: since the activity of the whole brain is higher than usual, the brain retains the pattern vividly for an extended amount of time.

up, when you think of tomorrow your frontal lobe fires up. When performing HAMR the effort required is no more strenuous than this.

Patterns Incorporating Patterns

The brain operates as a whole rather than as a group of individual structures or cells. The activity of one area of the brain affects the activity of the whole brain. Learning is something that occurs across the whole brain at once, not in any singular area.

The pattern on any given square (brain area) is a product of the input of all active squares.

In other words, if two active squares are connected together, each square will learn to produce a pattern that reflects the operations of both squares.

Two squares learn each other's patterns through **facilitation**. The left square does work that produces pattern **(L)**, and the right square does work that produces pattern **(F)**.

Each square learns the other square's pattern and produces its own pattern that incorporates both.

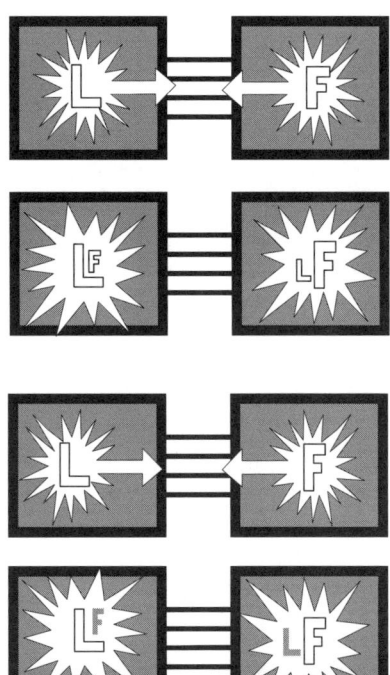

If squares communicate through **inhibition**:

Spheres of Thought. In the brain, evolution has produced a wiring configuration with specific criteria: survival, speed, and conservation of energy.

Aggregates

At any given moment there are many active areas in your brain. These areas operate at a distance from each other, but they operate as one. The pattern of activity on any region of cortex reflects its own activities along with the activities of every other operative region.

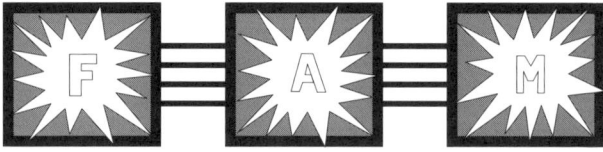

The activities of the left square produce pattern **(F)**, the center square produces pattern **(A)**, and the right square pattern **(M)**.

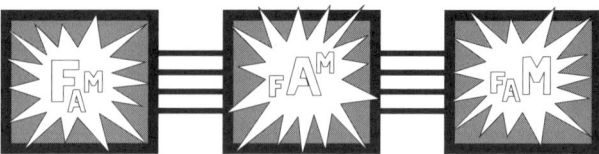

The pattern on each square favors its own activity, yet expresses the **aspects** of the others as well. The aggregate pattern for these squares contains aspects **(F),(M)** and **(A)**.

When many areas are contributing aspects to the aggregate pattern things can become complicated fast. To keep the clutter to a minimum, we simplify the aggregate pattern by assigning a new letter to it and showing it as that letter.

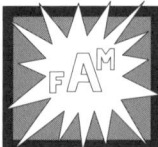 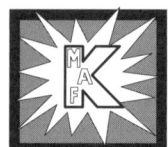 

Therefor, the sum of aspects **(F), (A) and (M)** is represented as **aggregate K**.

When we think of the future it is mentally out in front of us,

Frontal Lobes are the Staging Grounds of Complex Thought

Many areas of the neocortex have heavy tracts of fibers connecting them to the frontal lobes. These fibers carry a constant stream of information to and from the whole brain at once.

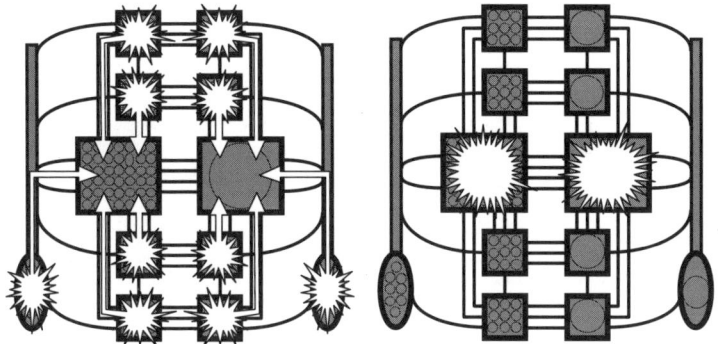

Left: information from the occipital lobes, parietal lobes, hippocampus, cingulate gyrus, and temporal lobes is sent to the frontal lobes.
Right: the frontal lobes integrate all of the information, along with other information for use in planning and thinking.

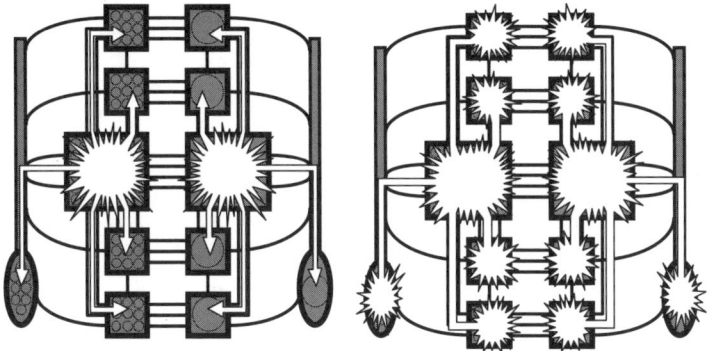

Left: the frontal lobes return the now modified information back to the respective areas, for reintegration into their own patterns.
Right: since everything is accomplished at once, the effect is that two huge patterns form (one across each side of the brain).

and when we think of the past it is back behind us. In terms of

Left-Brain Activity Combines into one Centralized Pattern: the X-aggregate

Each of the cerebral hemispheres has its own style of processing. The left hemisphere looks at things in a detail oriented manner and takes an aggressive approach to things.

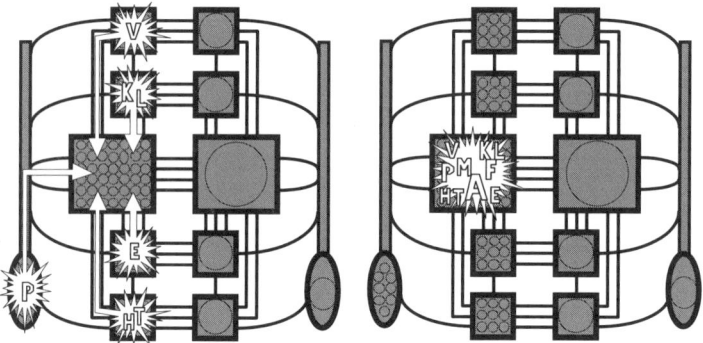

Left: patterns with information about vision(**V**), kinesthetic sensation(**K**), logic(**L**), memory(**P**), emotion(**E**), hearing(**H**) and tempo(**T**) are sent to the frontal lobes.
Right: the frontal lobes integrate all of the patterns, along with other information about planning(**F**) and motor programs(**M**), into the X-aggregate.

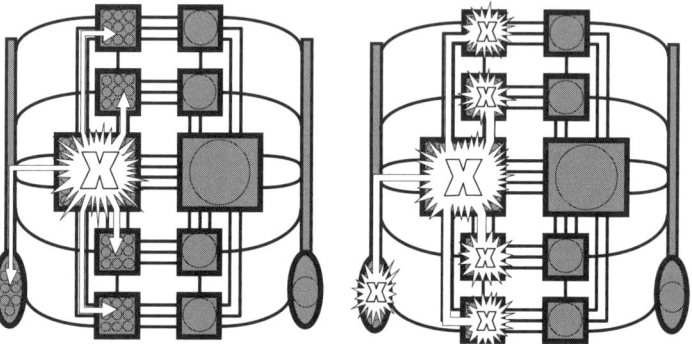

Left: the left frontal lobe returns the now integrated pattern to the other areas for reintegration into their own patterns.
Right: the left brain aggregate is a pattern that incorporates the activities of the entire left cerebral hemisphere.

the development of thought it makes sense that this would be the case. All complex animals have something in common, and

Right-Brain Activity Combines into one
Centralized Pattern: the Y-aggregate

The right hemisphere looks at things in a holistic manner, and takes a passive approach to things.

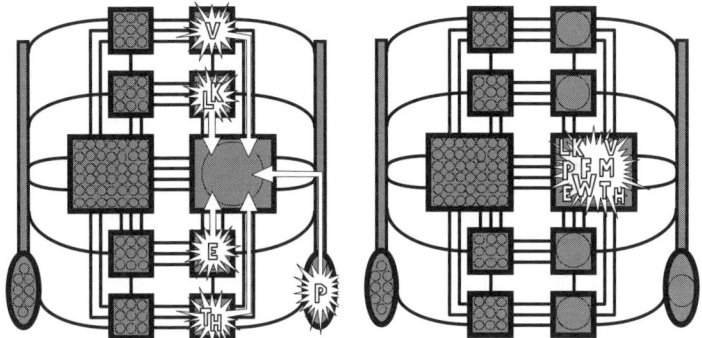

Left: patterns with information about vision**(V)**, kinesthetic sensation**(K)**, logic**(L)**, memory**(P)**, emotion**(E)**, hearing**(H)** and tempo**(T)** are sent to the frontal lobes.
Right: the right frontal lobe integrates all of the patterns along with other information about planning**(F)** and motor programs**(M)** into the Y-aggregate.

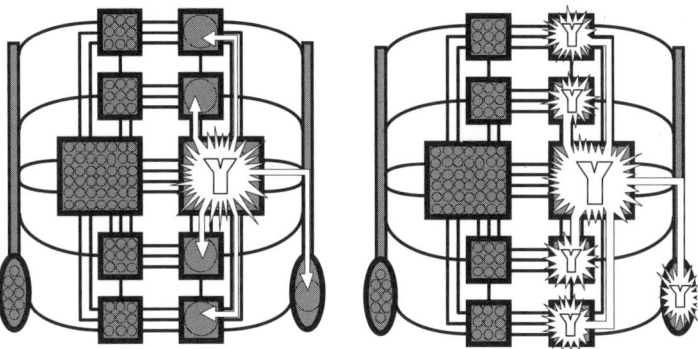

Left: the right frontal lobe returns the now integrated pattern to the other areas for reintegration into their own patterns.
Right: the right brain aggregate is a pattern that incorporates the activities of the entire right cerebral hemisphere.

that something is travel. The concept of time arises from this

Whole Brain Aggregate (Z)

With the right cerebral hemisphere hanging back and taking a cautious look at the world, the left cerebral hemisphere is ready to go on the offensive. Through inhibition, the two sides moderate (and remain appraised of) each other's activity. The result of this interaction is a balanced yet dynamic combination of solutions to life's challenges. The sum of all neurological action at any given time is called the "whole brain aggregate" or "Z aggregate."

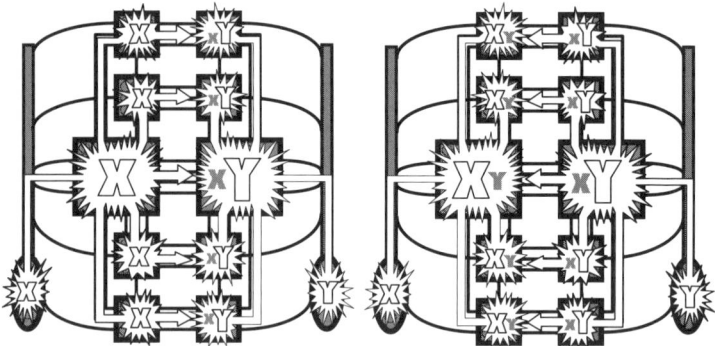

Left: left brain communicates to right brain through inhibition
Right: vice~versa

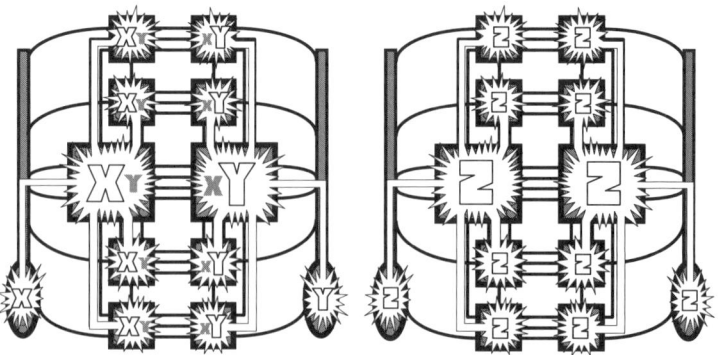

The combined efforts of both halves of the brain are expressed as one universal pattern **(Z)** .

simple activity.

The future is nothing more than that place to which we are going, and the past is nothing more than a place we have been. The organization of these two concepts in our minds is a result of the precedence of quick, effective retrieval in mental processing.

When traveling *to* a destination, our evolutionary forerunners were sometimes predisposed to contrive a strategy. When traveling *away from* an event our predecessors might have considered events that had just transpired. It does not stretch the

Beliefs

In an adult, situations are perceived through a system of filters that consist of right/wrong-codes, **beliefs**, and attitudes. Situations are dealt with through the employment of pre-learned motor patterns. Beliefs are depicted as arrows; positive beliefs are arrows pointing up, and negative beliefs are arrows pointing down.

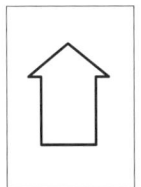 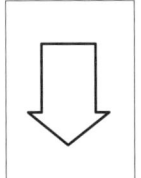

Positive Belief   **Negative Belief**

Different types of beliefs determine the effectiveness of various areas of the neocortex. Four types of beliefs that are of significant importance are beliefs that concern:

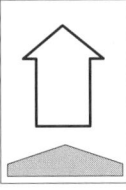 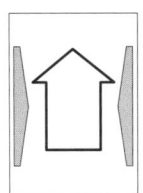 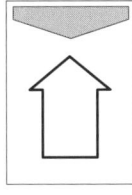 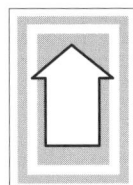

The Self   **Other People's Opinions**   **Super-natural Opinions**   **End Results**

imagination to see why past and future are mentally arranged as they are.

In primates and many other species of mammal the use of hands constitutes a huge percentage of time spent. Eating, grooming and, in higher primates, the use of tools require that the attention of an animal be fixed at the spatial location of the hands. Again, without taxing the imagination we may assume that many neurological connections are set to facilitate thought

Belief Systems

Belief systems assess a situation from all angles and help calculate the viability of reacting to it successfully.

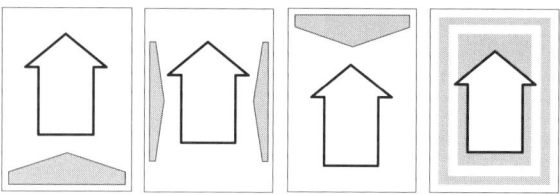

Motor or behavior patterns are facilitated by positive beliefs and inhibited by negative beliefs. Positive attitudes are facilitated by positive beliefs, and negative attitudes are facilitated by negative beliefs.

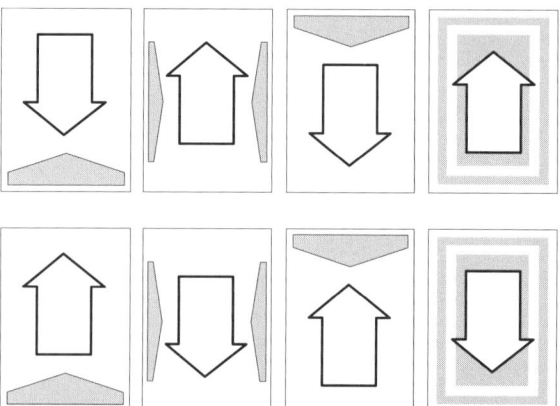

Belief systems can come in any combination of positive and negative beliefs.

in this area.

Many phrases in our language lend credence to this idea, and suggest an unconscious referral to neurological connections that may exist:

> "On the one hand I think this, but on the other hand I think that."
> "That idea might come in handy sometime."
> "Gotta hand it to you on that one."
> "Let us weigh the consequences."
> "Point out some possibilities."
> "Something is different, but I can't put my finger on it."
> "Get a hold of yourself."

All of these clauses and many more may help us to uncover the existence of useful neurological connections. It is already being established by researchers that speech and gesture[1] are produced by the same neurology. HAMR theory predicts that similar situations exist with respect to the convergence of

---

Attitudes and Behaviors

Attitudes are shown as triangles. Positive attitudes are depicted as triangles pointing up, and negative attitudes are depicted as triangles pointing down.

Positive Attitude

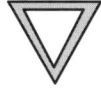

Negative Attitude

Behaviors (motor programs) are shown as the lightning-bolt symbol below. Motor programs that actively engage the environment (engagement behaviors) are pointing to the side, and motor programs that actively *avoid* engaging the environment (avoidance behaviors) are pointing down.

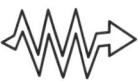

Engagement Behavior

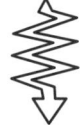

Avoidance Behavior

thought in the location of the hands. We theorize that the hands play a role in the processing of thoughts of all kinds (in primates).

Beliefs. Another interesting (albeit obscure) phenomenon is the ability of the cerebral hemispheres to maintain differing beliefs[2] or expectations. Each hemisphere is specialized for different aspects of thoughts or motor programs. However, the hemisphere most able to perform a task is not always the one that attempts to perform it. The hemisphere that thinks it can do a task will try, whether it actually can or not.

This concept may seem a little scary and bizarre, but with HAMR it can be made excellent use of. With respect to a given task, the steps taken for the HAMR process are used to make positive beliefs available to both hemispheres. The hemisphere most able to perform the task will then be predisposed to do so.

The Hebb Rule. Synapses connecting neurons that fire together become stronger if the collective activity is accompanied by a reward. What this means is that if a behavior works, it sticks. This principle holds true for everything from sex to rocket science. When the brain produces a pattern that brings about a reward, the synapses that make the pattern possible are strengthened.

Synapses that create patterns in the chaos are called Hebbian synapses. The synapses (and therefor the patterns) are sometimes reinforced by chemicals from the brain stem. The only ways that a pattern will be strengthened is if it produces a reward, occurs over and over, or occurs at a very high degree of excitation. In the event of the Hebb rule the brain stem decides what constitutes a "reward" and what does not.

A reward to the brain is something that produces endorphins. Some examples of reward are safety, orgasm, recognition, approval, nourishment, satisfaction, gratification, happiness, bliss, joy, contentment, comfort, relief, pleasure, and fulfillment. A pattern can be expected to stick if it produces one or more of these with an acceptable amount of energy expended.

In other words, if you have a pattern of activity on your neocortex that satisfies a need, your brain stem will produce and

Wheel of Hebb

Our brains are hard-wired by mother nature to pursue activities that bring about rewards. The Hebb Rule states that "connections between neurons that fire together become stronger if that firing is accompanied by a reward."

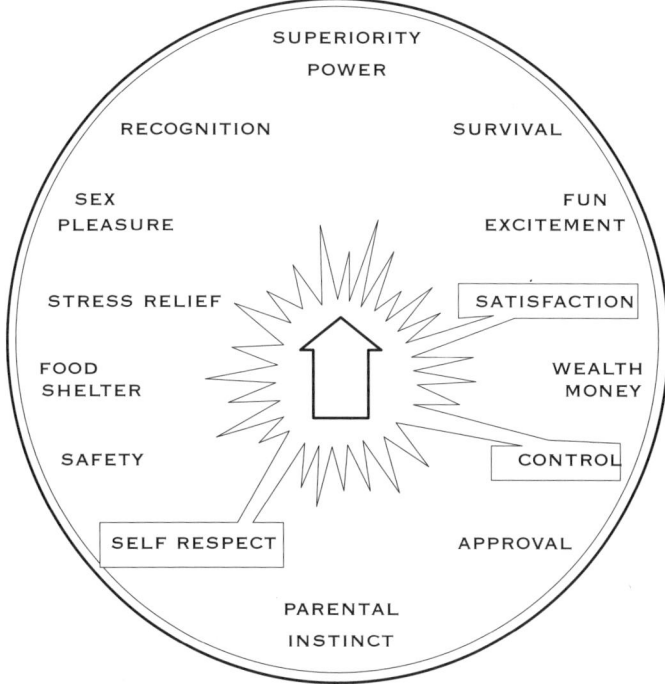

Some of the rewards that can bring about a strong neurological response (and result in learning) are listed here; they are referred to as **motives**.

The patterns being depicted on this wheel suggest that the positive belief in the center leads to rewards, in this case self respect, control and satisfaction. They are called **reward links**, because the pattern in the center is being linked to a *motive* or *reward*.

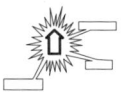

disperse chemicals that make that pattern stronger. The brain stem decides what a reward is, and it is the oldest and most primitive area of the brain. Knowing this makes it a fairly simple task to predict whether or not the brain will accept and strengthen a new pattern. If it gets results that favor the organism (you) in a substantial way, it will be permanent.

To get an idea of what this implies, consider the other name science uses to describe the brain stem: the "reptilian brain." It is called this because evolution sometimes works by building new structures right on top of the old ones.

Complex land creatures like mammals and birds evolved from reptiles. At the center of their neurology lurks the distant remnants of their past (the reptilian brain), still maintaining great power.

If you were to remove the huge cerebral hemispheres, and all the structures that support them, you would have roughly the same brain structure as a lizard. You could breathe, and your heart would beat. With round the clock care and spoon feeding you could stay alive for a long time.

If you were to remove the brain stem only and leave the rest of the brain you would be dead the instant it was disturbed. The brain stem is the one part of the brain without which there is no possibility of life. It is also the part of your brain that makes that most critical of decisions: which patterns of behavior will be saved, and which ones will be discarded.

The Hebb rule has been around for a good while and has been pretty well established. Chemicals from the brain stem cause patterns that are worthwhile to become solid and permanent. The goal of HAMR is to produce widespread cellular activity that is perceived by the brain stem to be advantageous, and thus worthy of such chemicals.

Gestalt. At any given moment in time your brain is tracking information about the present, comparing it to information about the past, and assessing how it will affect the future. This collection of activities is commonly referred to as a *gestalt*. For purposes of HAMR we assume that more neurons in the neocortex are utilized for the maintenance of a full gestalt than in any other mental activity. This principal proves its utility as well, and the HAMR Manual refers to it as **aggregates of activity** for a given situation.

Attitude and the Wheel of Hebb

For obvious reasons, positive attitudes can lead to many potential rewards. Negative attitudes can also lead to rewards if they keep you out of trouble.

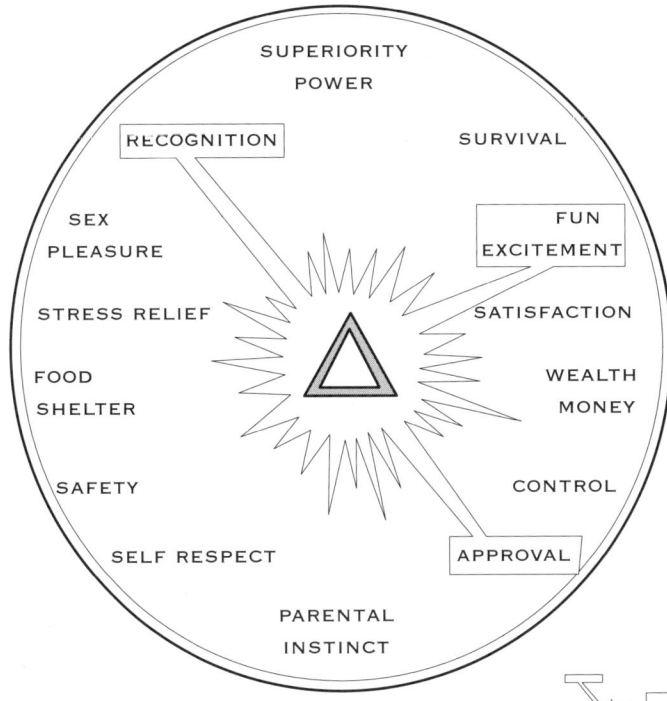

The **reward pattern** being derived here suggests that this positive attitude leads to self recognition, approval, fun and excitement.

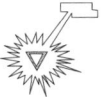

This negative attitude is linked to safety and/or survival.

The steps used to accomplish HAMR are designed to install new and better patterns of activity into a given aggregate. Patterns that prove useful to one aggregate will sometimes bleed over into others, but this cannot always be counted on. Each situation should be treated as being autonomous and receive individual attention.

The Hydraulic Model. The concept that emotions can somehow be "pent up" or "suppressed" has been with us for some time. Any emotion can be inhibited to some degree, but the one that seems to cause the most trouble is anger. Perfect understanding of the underlying processes involving anger still eludes science, but there are studies linking said "suppressed anger" to high blood pressure.[4]

HAMR theory adopts the *Hydraulic Model* for ease of explanation. For our purposes we will assume that anger can be suppressed, moderately expressed, or over-expressed.

According to Seymour Feshbach,

> "...there is substantial evidence that suppressed anger is linked to elevations in blood pressure, while frequently expressed anger is linked to coronary malfunctioning. However, the absence of anger is seen as having negative psychological consequences. Anger in moderation seems to be the ideal psychosomatic resolution."

Anger is one of the most important emotions, and it should be utilized to the greatest possible extent. This can only be accomplished when the entire brain is active in evoking and moderating it. A person who suppresses anger is actually limiting its influence to a small part of the brain (or perhaps a non-dominant hemisphere). This behavior uses vast amounts of energy and can only be sustained for a limited period of time. This is evident in cases of people who are sweet and timid right up until the moment they explode into uncontrollable fury. This is an unhealthy situation, and it is easily avoided by integrating anger into a more moderating influence by involving the whole brain.

Hemispheric Loss. Negative beliefs in a particular hemisphere result in partial or total loss of that hemisphere's cognitive function.

For example, if the right hemisphere believes that it cannot

Behavior and the Wheel of Hebb

Behavior is the means by which we interact with our environment. It is shaped by our perceptions, beliefs and the rewards that it brings.

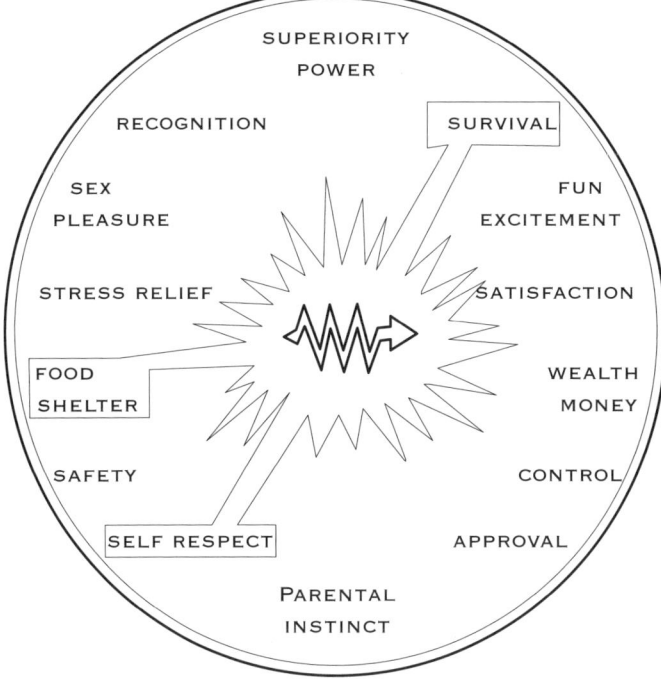

This **reward pattern** suggests that the behavior is motivated by survival, food, shelter, and self respect.

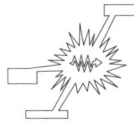

Avoidance behavior is often linked to safety and survival.

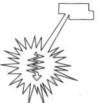

perform in a given situation, it will not. The result of this is a loss of global or holistic understanding. The right hemisphere looks at the big picture, and if a person does not see the whole

Right /Wrong Coding

Immersed in the chaos of thought patterns is a concept that stands on its own. It is the notion that some things are right and some things are wrong. Morality is the big Kahuna of mind; the neurological kingpen. Every cognitive thought pattern is regulated by codes that asses morality. This **right/wrong coding** applies to beliefs, attitudes, motives and behaviors, and it enjoys immense power.

Right   **Wrong**

Right coding is designated by a white star because it facilitates the pattern it applies to, and wrong coding is designated by a shaded star because it inhibits the pattern it applies to.

When you believe that what you are doing is right, you will be difficult, if not impossible, to stop.

When you believe that what you are doing is wrong, you will be filled with doubt and conflict and will be more easily dissuaded from your mission.

Right and wrong coding stands alone in that it supersedes all other types of patterns.

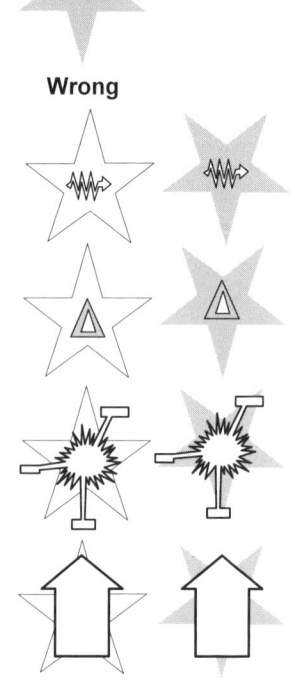

While wrong coding is a considerable force, it is not enough to stop patterns that achieve immediate and sizable rewards for the organism. People can still carry out behaviors that they feel are wrong, but the result may be depression and health problems associated with guilt and stress.

situation there will be a disproportionately large amount of detail-type thinking. Similarly, if the left hemisphere is lost a person will see only the big picture and will demonstrate a lack of effectiveness in dealing with details.

Both situations are completely undesirable. The best possible way to reason or think is with the full range of operational capability. This is *always* the case, even though a person with one or the other of these defects will believe otherwise. Fortunately, this irrational thought pattern will disappear when both hemispheres are enabled and can perform their respective functions.

The Wish. A wish is a long-standing desire under pressure. The mental experience of a wish is very deep. That is because a lot of neurons are involved with the desire that is being suppressed. The neurology that is involved with a wish is widespread and diverse. It also takes a lot of neurons to keep a wish inhibited.

For this reason, letting a wish loose has one of the most powerful effects that can be achieved by HAMR. When coupled with right-coding, positive beliefs, positive attitudes, behaviors and motives, nothing can stop a wish. In the immortal words of Jimminy Cricket, "When you wish upon a star your dreams come true."

A wish may be called a "true desire," and once loose there is no putting it back. If your dreams are to do something worthwhile for mankind, then do us all a favor and go for it. The rain forests are being decimated, the ozone layer is being depleted, and the outlook for the human race is bleak. If you have a wish to do something that will improve our collective situation, let it loose. The world needs you, and to be happy you probably have no other choice.

Energy levels. One of the prime decision making criterion of the brain stem is how much energy is necessary to produce a given reward. Since the brain stem has the chemicals, it gets to make the decisions. The criterion on which it bases its logic is *results*.

It takes more energy (and produces less success) for the brain to do a task with the incorrect cerebral hemisphere than it does to use the correct one. We can therefore predict that if someone is attempting to perform a task with the wrong side of his or her

---

Situational Programs

The brain assesses and responds to individual situations. It filters incoming information through moral-coding and the belief system, devises strategy based on the prevailing attitude, and acts through behavior and/or motor patterns. The **situational program** is the control-panel of the brain.

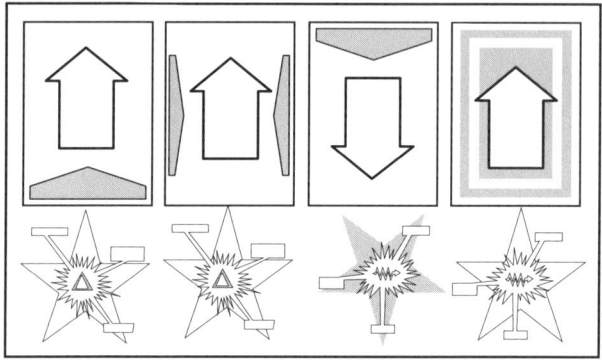

A program consists of a belief system, some attitudes, some behaviors, and right and wrong coding supporting or inhibiting each one. Attitudes and behaviors are shown with their respective reward patterns(motives) and right/wrong codes.

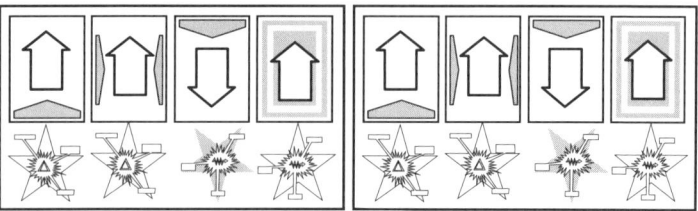

Essentially, the neocortex consists of two brains, and each one perceives and responds to the world differently. Each cerebral hemisphere adds its unique processing skill to the conglomerate of thought, and each one maintains its own discreet set of programs. When both programs match or agree with each other, there can be well-coordinated effort between the hemispheres.

brain, he or she is using too much energy. Introducing a pattern which includes both sides will provide the option to be more successful and use less energy. This is something the brain stem can understand, and endorphins will be the inevitable result.

Recreating the Big Scare. The frontal lobes accommodate

Situational Programs Govern the Activities of the X and Y aggregates

For each situation, both sides of the brain maintain discreet programs that manage their operations. These situational programs govern the activities of the cerebral hemispheres.

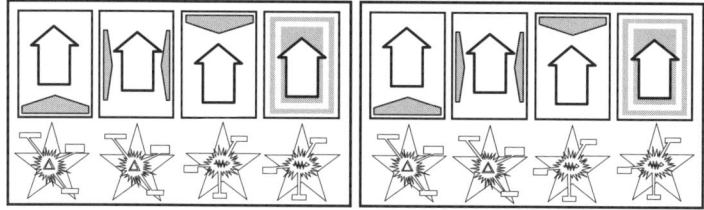

In this hypothetical situation both programs are of sterling quality with 100% positive beliefs, positive attitudes and behavioral patterns that are linked to substantial rewards.

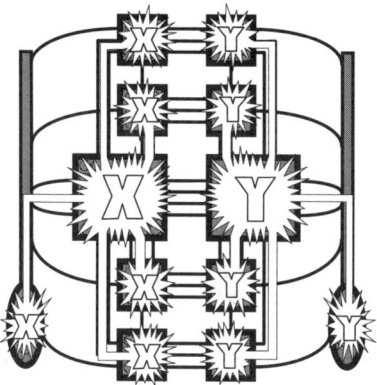

The result of this combination is two fully active hemispheres that share and work towards the same goals with equal enthusiasm. These are perfect neurological conditions for success. With HAMR, the goal toward which you strive is to duplicate these conditions with respect to every important situation in your life.

the staging grounds of the imagination. All of the lobes of the brain are wired directly into these largest of lobes. The areas that are known to produce language, gesture, and planning are

Negativity

Negative beliefs and attitudes have no place in situations where engagement with the environment and a positive outcome are necessary. The programs below have only negative beliefs, bad attitudes, avoidance behavior and *wrong coding*. A brain with this setup has no chance of success, and its neurological level of activity will reflect it.

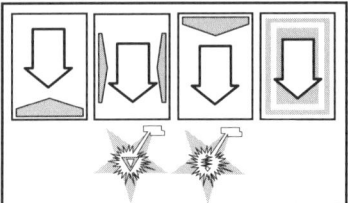 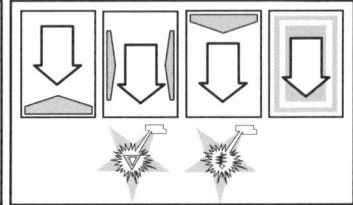

If the situation these programs address is something dangerous like *lion-taming* or *razor-blade-swallowing,* then they are entirely appropriate. If the situation is *dealing with other people,* it would not be an advantageous combination in any sense.

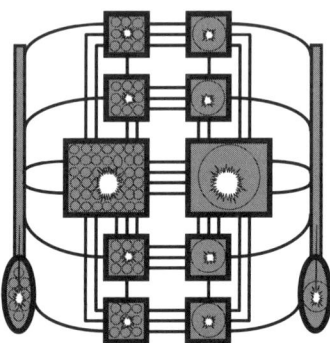

The result of the above programs is two relatively inactive hemispheres that work only towards avoiding the situation. Sometimes the hemispheres will have positive programs on one side and negative programs on the other. When this occurs there will be an activity-deficit in the anterior frontal lobe that has the negative program, and a personality that flips back and forth between two extremes.

located here. Therefore, the theoretical objective of HAMR is to "print" new and more useful patterns of activity on the frontal lobes.

The way we do that is to recreate "the big scare" (excessive cerebral activity brought on by trauma and resulting in strengthened patterns) through superior numerical force. Areas of cortex stimulate each other, and the frontal lobes receive excitation from all areas of the neocortex. The theory is that exciting the targeted areas of cortex simultaneously will cause the new pattern to be spread to critical areas of the brain and stimulate the brainstem to release pattern-reinforcing chemicals.

Justification. When a pattern has been selected by the brain stem to be strengthened, the rest of the brain will automatically seek to justify it with "rationalization" or "logic". Finding justification helps the pattern to be smoothly integrated into the overall state of mind with the minimum possible amount of mental friction. The parietal and frontal lobes are most likely involved in this aspect of the operation.

As time passes the brain finds more reward and fuller justification, and the new pattern becomes ever stronger. People think that they are logical and that their thoughts and motivations are high and pure. The truth is that we are all puppets on the strings of a reptile brain.

This is not a bad thing, and realizing it can even lead to a bit of table-turning. Knowing how your brain really works will enable you to call the shots yourself, and logic can take a big step forward. The evolution of the human mind can march on.

Ideal Brain Conditions. They say that people use about ten percent of their brain capacity. If you could bring about full mental function, or one hundred percent usage, you would be operating under "ideal brain conditions". This theoretically perfect state is the overall goal toward which you strive with the HAMR system.

Adding brain power is always better than subtracting it. You can never go wrong if you stick to a basic philosophy of adding only positive things to your mind. So be liberal with installing good thoughts and concepts and avoid negative ones like the plague. Positive beliefs add brain power, and negative beliefs

---

Spatial Locations of Thought

The brain has evolved spatial thought processes that utilize spatial areas around the body. The future is located out in front of us, the past is behind us, and the area immediately in front of and surrounding our body is the present. The present is divided into two areas which represent associated and disassociated meaning.

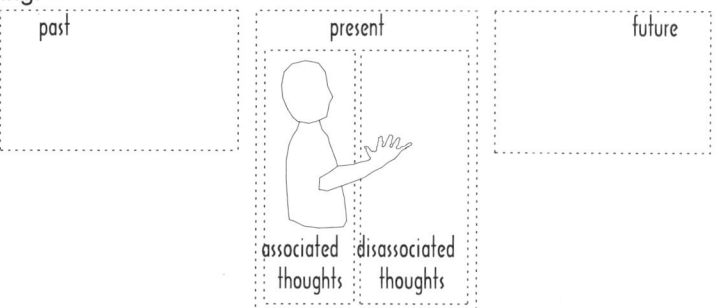

The disassociated areas are split into two distinct theaters of mental operation. One is for either side of the brain. These areas are the place where ideas come together and information is manipulated into various forms.

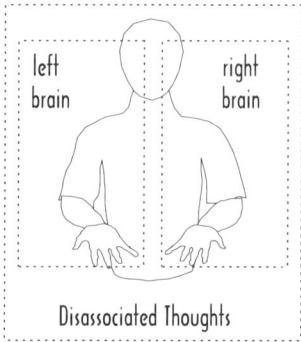

There is evidence that the hands play a part in some mental processing, and these are the spheres of thought where this is likely to occur. It is these *staging grounds of the imagination* that you will utilize in carrying out your pattern-installation.

subtract brain power. Smart is always better; and more brain is always better than less brain.

The Imagination

The imagination is a place where the brain does trial runs of situations. Sometimes it is used as an escape to a mental place where things feel better. Ideas in the imagination spheres are considered to be not real and disassociated. For HAMR the real advantage of the imagination is its ability to simulate non-existing conditions without interference from the learned aggregates.

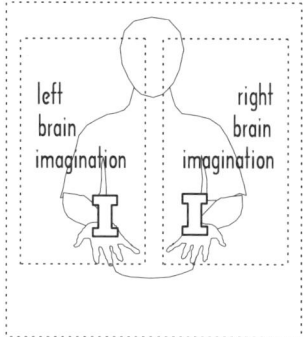 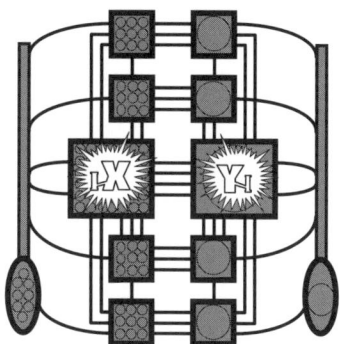

We assume that the frontal lobes contain much of the circuitry responsible for imagination **(I)**.

Associated thoughts that belong to the aggregates must conform to the rules in the situational programs. If they do not conform to the rules, they will be rejected by the aggregates. As an example: when someone important to you dies your brain will vigorously combat accepting the loss and will require much adjustment to feel comfortable once again.

Conditions that are rejected by the brain can be simulated in a disassociated state, then installed directly into the aggregates using the hammer.

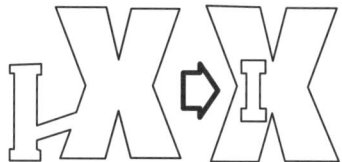

To simulate non-existing conditions, you simply accept the fact that what you are imagining (in your hand) is not true, it is merely *being imagined*. This effectively bypasses any mental barriers. From the safety of your own imagination you can fantasize anything you wish, and your mind is powerless to stop you.

Perceptions of different types are made possible by different areas of the brain. Occipital lobes allow perception of sight, parietal lobes allow perception of touch, olfactory cortex allows perception of smell, etc.

Other perceptions may be more subtle and selective. Some people with great qualities are unable to perceive their goodness. This is called low self esteem, and it is debilitating. In principle, you could think of low self esteem as the inability to utilize areas of the brain that perceive self worth.

OPO-Other People's Opinions. A powerful force in the brain of human beings is the expectations of other human beings. We crave the attention, interaction and approval of others. These things are of paramount importance, and they affect our behavior in many ways. Good or bad, people tend to do what is expected of them, so it follows that the opinions of others are a strong motivator that utilizes substantial amounts of cerebral cortex.

Many of our unconscious behaviors are brought about by what we believe others think. Do not underestimate the importance of this concept, for it proves to be very useful in the practice of HAMR.

Supernatural Opinions. The notion of a higher and more authoritative power has, for whatever reason, evolved to be a powerful influence in the neurology of Homo Sapiens. People often feel strongly about a religious figure or cause. When installing patterns dealing with supernatural opinions, tailor them to your own particular religious preference.

The issue of whether or not a god actually exists is utterly irrelevant. What is poignantly obvious is that it *does* matter what a person *feels* or *believes* to be the truth. For this reason, HAMR is designed to take full advantage of the situation. Your personal belief about what a god might be like, or if one even exists, will not affect the outcome of the process. You can be a full blown atheist and still take advantage of the "neurology of god." All you have to do is follow the steps.

In this book the neurology of supernatural opinions is utilized in a variety of situations. Once you understand what it does you can tailor it to fit your individual wants and needs. The primary uses that will be outlined herein are with respect to health, happiness, and success. Other uses will no doubt suggest themselves to you as you go along. The process is simple and easy, and it will work regardless of your convictions.

Effects. The effects of HAMR are bizarre, and nothing less than miraculous. The personality changes in ways that are spectacular to others but almost imperceptible you. Satisfaction comes in a roundabout manner. It will seem as if the rest of the world has changed its attitude toward you.

The first few days or weeks after a change are sometimes miserable and difficult. That is because you are no longer willing to accept less than what you want. The world must learn how to deal with you in a fresh, new way, and it tends to resist change. However, after proving that you can succeed at what you desire to do or have, life gets used to providing what you demand, and a feeling of deep satisfaction begins to take hold. Once this satisfaction is experienced, you can never go back to living without it.

In summary, the human mind is the result of complex electro-chemical interactions in the brain. Knowing how it works can suggest a course of action for reprogramming it. Many areas in the brain support individual patterns of activity that combine to form complex thought. When thoughts that produce a reward occur, the brain stem secretes chemicals that reinforce them.

The goal of the HAMR system is to produce useful patterns of activity across the surface of the entire cerebral hemispheres. These patterns should initially exist with a high degree of vigorousness and should provide substantial reward. In the next chapter we examine the steps for installing such patterns.

---

[1]Palmer Morrel-Samuals and Robert M. Krauss, Columbia University, *Word Familiarity Predicts Temporal Asynchrony of Hand Gestures and*

Speech Journal of Experimental Psychology: Learning, Memory, and Cognition 1992 (Vol. 18, No.3, 615-622)

[2]J. Levy and C. Trevarthen *"Metacontrol of Hemispheric function in Splitbrain Patients"* Journal of Experimental Psychology: Human Perception and Performance 2 1976 (299-312)

[3]Joel E. Dimsdale, MD, Chester Pierce, MD, David Schoenfeld, PhD, Anne Brown, RN, Randall Zuzman, MD, and Robert Graham, MD. *Suppressed Anger and Blood Pressure: The Effects of Race, Sex, Social Class, Obesity, and Age.* Psychosomatic Medicine Vol. 48, No. 6 (July/August 1986)

[4]Seymour Feshbach, University of California-Los Angeles, *Reconceptualizations of Anger: Some Research Perspectives* Journal of Social and Clinical Psychology (Vol. 4, No. 2, 1986, pp. 123-132)

4

The Hammer

The steps that are used to execute HAMR are fondly referred to as "the hammer." Only requiring a few seconds to accomplish, it is easily preformed by anyone. It is simple, fast, and easy to do. *Do not underestimate its power.* It only takes one repetition to modify your behavior and start your brain down a new trail of thought. Once the hammer has been performed there is no way to reverse it.

There is already much evidence to suggest that HAMR has great promise as a self help device, and that it will demonstrate itself to have application in treating serious emotional disorders.

As mentioned in chapter one, *be sure to carefully study all of the HAMR diagrams before perusing the text.* This will enhance your understanding of the process and allow you to place the information in its proper perspective.

Overview. The hand motions used for HAMR are based on a simple series of actions that have been around for a long time and have been used in several different contexts. Its most recent usage has been in the field of Neuro Linguistic Programming, where it is recognized as the *visual squash* and *the conflict integration model.*

The visual squash was mentioned by Bandler and Grinder[1] in the late 1970's, as a method of integrating multiple personalities. It was executed by imagining a personality in each hand and then smashing them together. It was said that if the person was lucky the personalities would come back apart on their own.

Bob Dilts contrived a cleaner[2] and much more effective way of using the movements. He calls it the "conflict integration model," and it seems to work pretty well. Many a person has benefited from this adaptation. Used to resolve psychological conflict, the methodology is to place one side of a mental disagreement in each hand, then negotiate them into compatible forms of thought before combining them. It is described in a book called <u>Beliefs, Pathways to Health and Well Being</u>.

HAMR uses the hand motions with a little bit different slant

Your Mission

The goal you work towards with HAMR is to decide which situations you want or need to succeed in, then make sure that **both** sides of your brain have:

> *all four types of *positive beliefs*
> *at least one *positive attitude* linked to at least one *reward*
> *at least one *positive behavior* linked to at least one *reward*
> *right coding* on all of the above

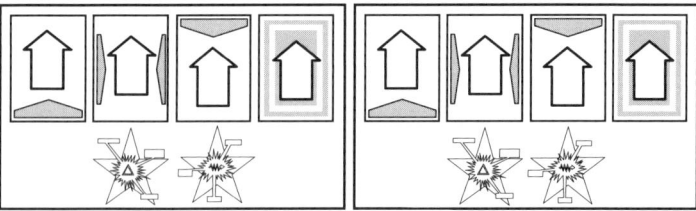

To produce positive programs like the ones above, new patterns are installed with *the <u>hammer</u>*.

on things. No attempt is made to appease the Brain God by securing some kind of mental "permission" from yourself. Your brain belongs to you the same way your foot does. It serves at your pleasure, and you have every right to maximize its perfor-

Installing New Patterns

New patterns are placed on the frontal lobes, then installed into one side of the brain at a time. The new pattern to be installed will simulate conditions that would exist if things *actually were* different.

To place a pattern on the frontal lobe, you imagine that it is in your hand as the drawing depicts. The pattern being installed is called the new pattern(**N**). A new pattern is always an imaginary depiction of what life would be like with *new conditions*. The hand holding the new pattern is called the *new hand*.

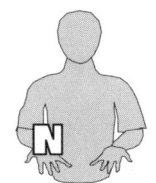

The other hand contains conditions as they currently exist and it is referred to as the *old hand*. Simply thinking of the situation you are working on will stimulate the old pattern(**O**) to fire up.

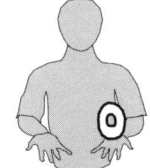

Every time a new pattern is installed into the brain, the hammer is performed twice: once with the new hand on the left and the old hand on the right and once with the new hand on the right and the old hand on the left.

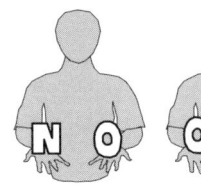 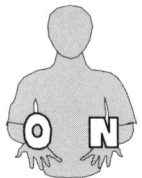

New patterns to install consist of the four types of beliefs, attitudes, motives, behaviors and right/ wrong codes.

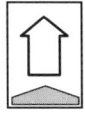 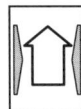 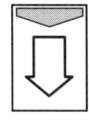 

  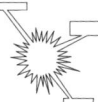

The H.A.M.R. Manual

mance to the largest possible extent.

HAMR represents a new way of thinking about psychology. It goes against many traditional superstitions about the mind. Yet, out with the old and in with the new. No doubt one day

---

Creating Mental Scenarios

The pattern in the *new* hand is an imaginary scenario of what life with the improved thought pattern would be like. As an example, the following descriptions will apply to the situation of *doing the hammer*.

 Right/wrong codes: installing a **right** pattern about *doing the hammer:* in the new hand imagine what it would be like if doing the hammer is right in every sense.

 Positive beliefs about the self: installing a **belief** that *you are naturally good at doing the hammer:* in the new hand imagine what it would be like if you were the kind of person that is naturally good at doing the hammer.

 Positive beliefs about outside opinions: installing a **belief** that *everybody knows that you are naturally good at doing the hammer:* in the new hand imagine what it would be like if everybody knew that you were the kind of person that is naturally good at doing the hammer.

 Positive beliefs about supernatural opinions: installing a **belief** that *supernatural beings expect you to be good at doing the hammer.* In the New hand, imagine what it would be like if some religious figure or supernatural force expected you to succeed wildly with HAMR.

 Positive beliefs about the outcome: installing a belief that you will succeed wildly with HAMR: In the New hand, imagine what it would be like if you actually were going to succeed wildly with HAMR.

 Attitudes: installing an attitude that you will succeed wildly with HAMR: In the New hand, imagine what it would be like if you had the attitude that you are going to succeed with HAMR no matter what.

 Behaviors: installing a behavior that will make you succeed wildly with HAMR: In the New hand, imagine what it would be like if you were the kind of person that aggressively works to master HAMR.

 Motives: linking the aforementioned behavior to superiority: In the New hand, imagine what it would be like if doing well with HAMR would actually make you superior to everyone else.

HAMR will be displaced by a more effective system, but for now, there is much to be learned about this one.

This book attempts to divulge information that has shown itself to be reliable and capable of attaining positive results. Much trial and error has gone into the formation of this system. For you, learning how to use it will be a similar process. HAMR is a collection of tools that must be mastered, but once mastered will be with you always. When you have it as a constant companion you can tailor it instantly to augment your development in any situation.

Superior Numerical Force. The HAMR system is an attempt to achieve two outcomes:

#1 integrate new and useful patterns of activity across large areas of the cerebral cortex, and

#2 light up the frontal lobes so brightly that the new and useful patterns become strengthened.

Both of these outcomes are achieved at the same time with the hammer. It is accomplished by merging patterns from all over the brain into a single pattern while raising the brain's excitation level high enough to burn it into permanence. The way we attempt this is through utilizing a superior numerical force of neurons acting on other neurons.

As pointed out in the chapter on the brain, some neurons excite each other, and some inhibit each other. For bringing the brain to a higher activity level, neurons that we now consider are the groups that use primarily excitation to communicate to other groups. We turn our attention to them in an attempt to explain the effects of the hammer. The theory goes something like this:

Patches of neurons excite other patches of neurons that are connected to them. Some patches of neurons are connected to many other patches. Normally the groups only excite each other to a certain degree, but if an area is connected to several other areas that all become excited at once, it will become intensely active. This extra high intensity should be enough to cause strengthening of a given pattern of activity.

For example, let us assume that groups of neurons can have

Condensed Hammer

The hammer is a sequence of thoughts and hand motions that is used to install new mental patterns into the whole brain at once (aggregates). First a pattern is placed on one frontal lobe and a series of maneuvers expands it while bringing the neocortex to a higher-than-normal state of excitation; then the new pattern is forced into an associated state. The hammer should always be performed twice, installing the new pattern into both cerebral hemispheres (the X and Y aggregates).

#1 Consider the situation you wish to change. The X and Y-aggregates (old patterns) for that situation will automatically pop into their respective sides.

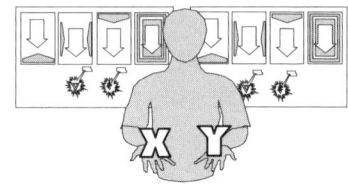

#2 Imagine on one hand a new pattern(**N**) to be installed and in the other hand the old pattern(**O**).

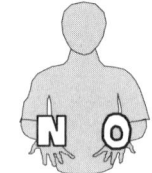

#3 Have the contents of the new hand(**N**) look at the contents of the old hand(**O**), then have the contents of the old hand(**O**) look at the contents of the new hand(**N**).

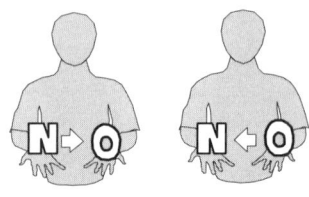

#4 Imagine the past(**P**) being in one hand, then the other.

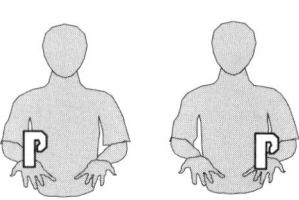

degrees of activity on a scale of one to ten. At one the neurons

#5 Imagine the future**(F)** being in one hand, then the other.

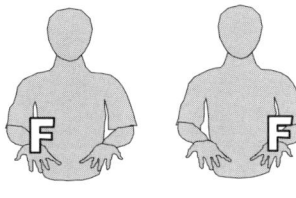

#6 Imagine the present [everything you can see**(V)**, hear**(H)**, and feel**(K)** around you at the time] being in one hand, then the other.

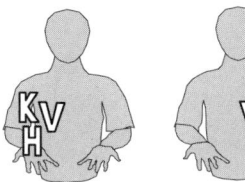

#7 Combine the two sides into a mixture**(M)**.

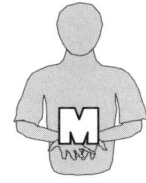

#8 Smash the mixture into your chest.

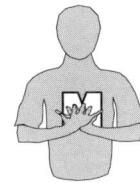

#9 Repeat steps 1-8, beginning with the new pattern**(N)** in the other hand.
Since the hammer may bring the

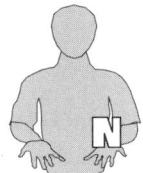

brain to a higher than normal activity level, there is reason to believe that a higher than normal amount of strengthening may occur to the new pattern. However, this strengthening will only supply the new pattern with enough of a boost to get started, and permanence will ultimately be decided by the Hebb rule.

are at rest, gently firing chaotic, perhaps meaningless patterns. At five the neurons are firing heavily, and out of the chaos come patterns that have meaning. Above nine the neurons are so excited that the brain stem secretes chemicals which strengthen any patterns that are present.

Under these terms, imagine that a master group of one thousand neurons is connected to three other slave groups that also contain one thousand neurons each. If one of the slave groups becomes excited to a level five, the master group also achieves a level five. If two of the slave groups become excited to a level five, the master group becomes active to a level seven. But if all three of the slave groups become excited to a level five, the master group is activated to a level nine and is furiously excited. The brain stem detects level nine activity and secretes chemicals that strengthen the patterns of activity on *all four groups*.

The new pattern that has been burned into the master and slave groups is now strong and can easily be fired up by the brain. It is still possible, however, for the pattern to be rejected or *forgotten*. In fact, this will happen naturally to some degree unless the brain continues to strengthen and expand the new connections.

That is where the Hebb rule comes in. As previously men-

Note

Do the steps quickly. Large amounts of concentration are not necessary or even desirable. The idea is to think of the past, present, and future only long enough to fire up the targeted areas of cortex.. Specific memories or plans are irrelevant. Wasting time on concentration only gives the targeted areas time to lose their excitation. The whole process should take only about thirty seconds or less.

Keep your eyes open. One large and valuable area of the brain is the occipital lobes. Closing your eyes lessens the number of neurons that are participating.

tioned, the Hebb rule states that connections between neurons that fire together will become strengthened if the firing is accompanied by a reward.

We may therefore complete the scenario with Hebb. The slave and master groups are firing along quietly when one slave group has a great idea and fires up to level five, followed immediately by the second and third groups. The master group participates in the idea and is ignited to first level five, then seven, then explodes into level nine. The brain stem releases chemicals, and the new idea becomes strong across all four groups. Over

---

Expanded Hammer
Step 1

The first thing to do is light up the patterns that control the situation you are about to work on. Just thinking about a situation will activate the patterns, making them available for modification.

#1 Consider the situation you wish to change. The X and Y-aggregates (old patterns) for that situation will automatically pop into their respective sides.

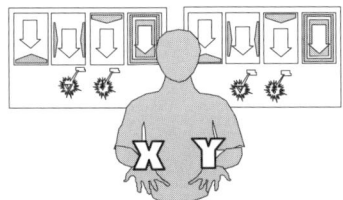

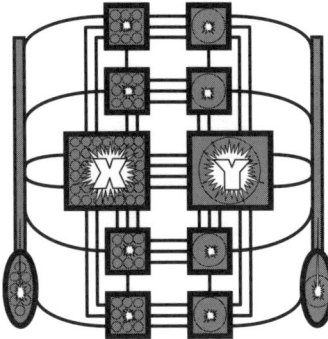 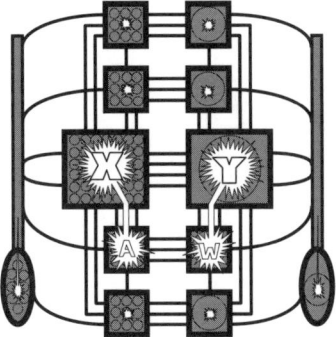

The X and Y-aggregates light up on the frontal lobes, then the cingulate gyrus on either side becomes excited with its respective array of emotion (approach versus withdrawal).

time the brain discovers that the new pattern or idea brings about a reward. The Hebb rule is invoked, and the new pattern grows stronger by growing more connections to support it.

This series of events is the goal of HAMR. The steps that follow are designed to establish new and more useful patterns of activity across large portions of the cerebral hemispheres.

The mind can only concentrate on one thing at a time, but it can move rapidly from one thought to another. Once an area of cortex is excited it will remain that way for several seconds. By

Expanded Hammer
Step 2

The second thing to do is light up the new pattern on the left-frontal lobe. The new pattern should consist of an imaginary scene that depicts what life would be like with the new belief, attitude or motor program that is being installed.

#2 Imagine on one hand a new pattern(**N**) to be installed, and in the other hand the old pattern(**O**). Since the aggregates of a par-

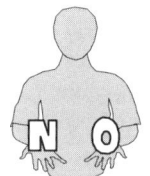

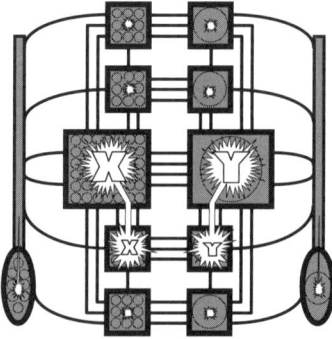
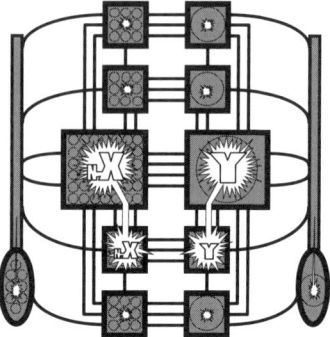

ticular situation have been evoked(**left**), the new pattern *joins* the X-aggregate, albeit in a disassociated state.

thinking a particular thought you can activate a slave group. Then you can move your attention to another slave group, then another. If your thoughts move to the second and third groups before the first one has time to fade, the master group will achieve a blistering level nine.

The brain is comprised of groups of neurons that are connected together in various ways. Looking at the Diagram of

Expanded Hammer
Step 3

Through inhibition, the left and right brain aggregates merge activity. The new pattern is spread from one frontal lobe to the other, after which it is ready to be burned into place.

#3 Have the contents of the new hand(**N**) look at the contents of the old hand(**O**), then have the contents of the old hand(**O**) look at the contents of the new hand(**N**).

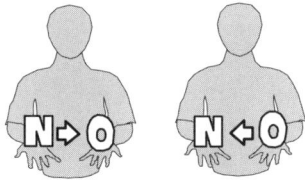

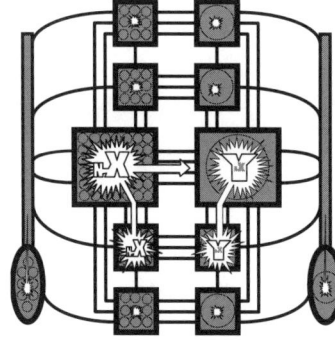
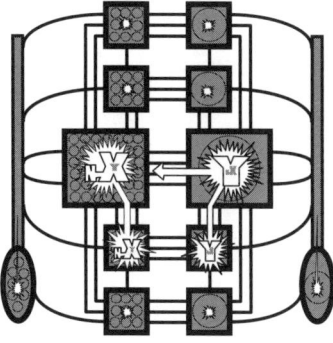

The new pattern becomes a part of both sides of the brain, but in a different way. The left brain integrates the new pattern into its activities by using it to reconstruct its facilitory action, and the right brain integrates the new pattern into its activities through the inhibitory shadow of what the other side is doing. After the pattern has been "burned in" this way, the roles will be reversed, and pattern will be burned in again. In this way both sides of the brain will be endowed with facilitory and inhibitory action that strive for the same end.

HAMR, you will observe that the frontal lobes are wired directly to several very large areas of cerebral cortex. The frontal lobes are the *master* groups, and the rest of the lobes are the *slave* groups. The will alone can only excite the slave lobes to a

Expanded Hammer
Step 4

To involve the hippocampus (and other areas involved with memory), simply think back to the first memory that pops to mind and imagine that it is in one hand, then the other.

#4 Imagine the past(**P**) being in one hand, then the other.

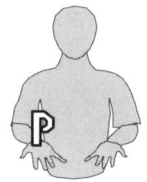 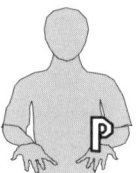

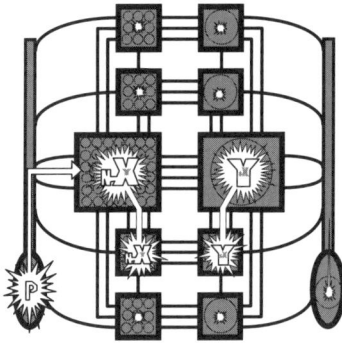 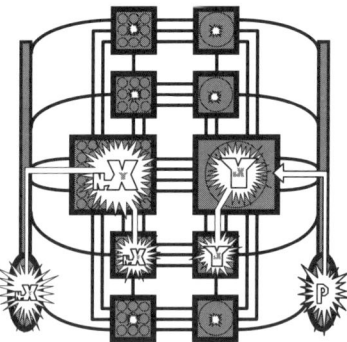

Each hippocampus activates its version of a memory that will adequately stimulate it. As each one is activated the aggregate containing the new pattern spreads into it.

It does not matter what memory is used. The object is to stimulate areas of the brain, not a particular memory.

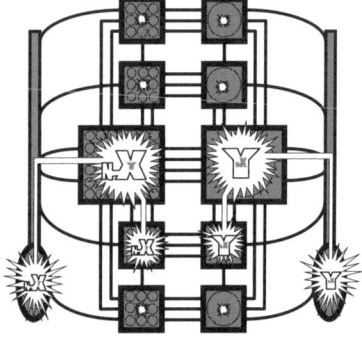

certain degree, not enough to burn in patterns. However, if all the areas connected to the frontal lobes become excited at once, they will participate in raising the level of activity. Enough excitement can be achieved to push this action "over the top," and

Expanded Hammer
Step 5

The frontal lobes process much of the information used in planning for the future. To light up the frontal areas that do this work, simply thinking forward to any future period of time will do.

#5 Imagine the future(**F**) being in one hand, then the other.

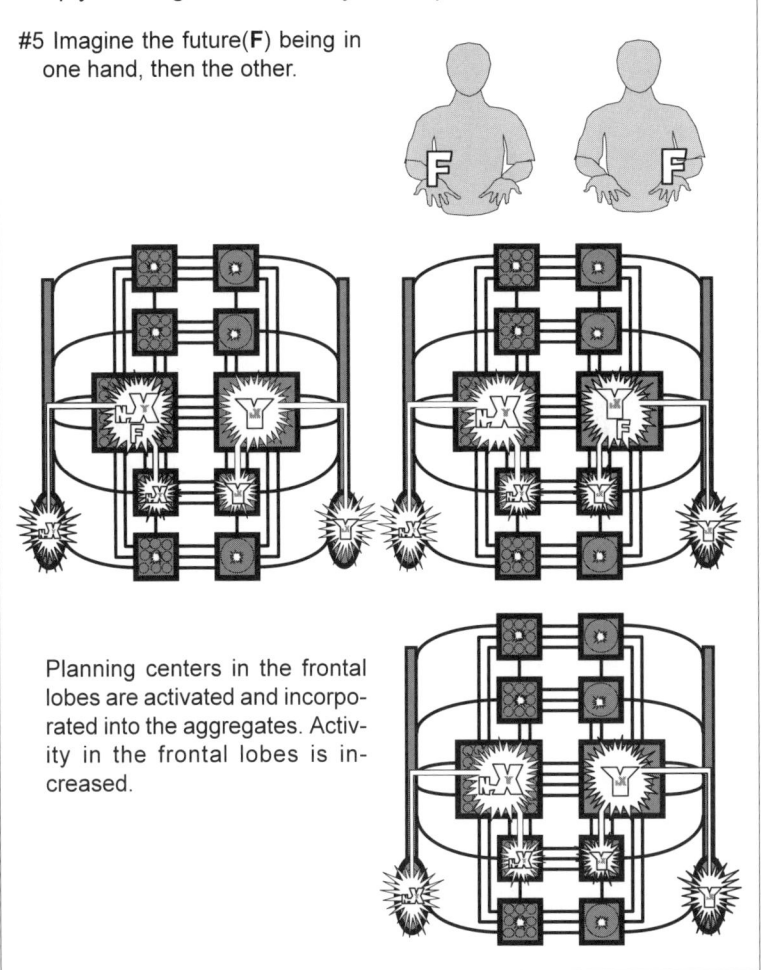

Planning centers in the frontal lobes are activated and incorporated into the aggregates. Activity in the frontal lobes is increased.

the brain stem will secrete pattern-reinforcing chemicals.

Some areas can be activated by the will, and some cannot. The will is capable of firing groups of neurons to a certain level of activity and no more. The level of activity that can be achieved

Expanded Hammer
Step 6

Activation of the occipital lobes, parietal lobes, and temporal lobes brings them into the aggregates and finishes lighting up the brain.

#6 Imagine the present [everything you can see(**V**), hear(**H**), and feel(**K**) around you at the time] being in one hand, then the other. As the remaining areas of cor-

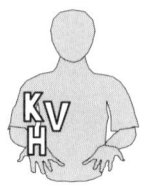
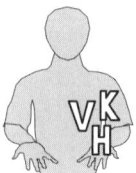

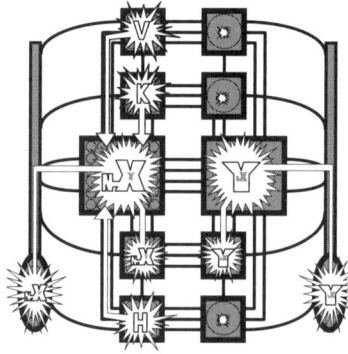
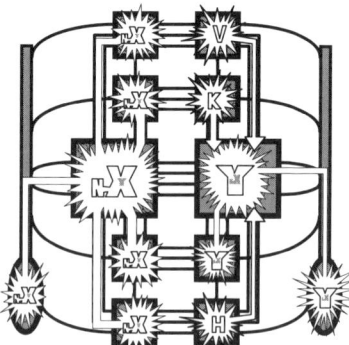

tex are activated they supply patterns that support the aggregates. The new pattern has now been spread to the left brain in a facilitory form, and to the right brain in an inhibitory form. It remains in a disassociated state.

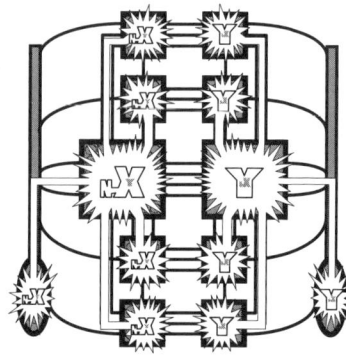

through will power alone is not generally enough to significantly strengthen a new pattern (except with sheer repetition, which has only a marginal effect). Other factors must intervene if this is to occur.

The goal of the hammer is to use the will to induce a pattern of activity on a particular area of cortex, then fire up the major areas that connect to them. The way we produce this effect is by quickly directing the will in several different neurological directions for just long enough to bring them to a good solid activity level. These directions consist of the past, present and future. Theoretically this will trick the brainstem into secreting

---

Expanded Hammer
Step 7

Placing one hand underneath the other forces the two patterns into a mixture. The two cerebral hemispheres must conceive of the left and right patterns as one pattern that occupies the same space and time.

#7 Combine the two sides into a mixture(**M**).

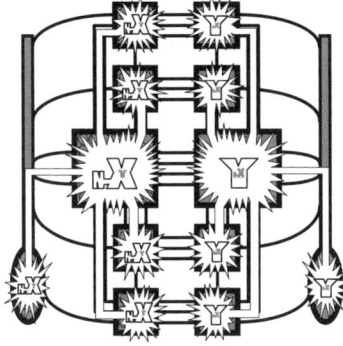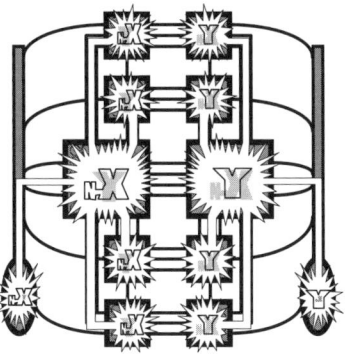

Sometimes at this point the person doing the hammer feels a slight swelling sensation at the front of their head.

chemicals that strengthen patterns. Thus the term "superior numerical force." Another way to look at it is *reproducing the big scare* with a positive outcome.

It is an oversimplification to think that the brain works ex-

---

Expanded Hammer
Step 8

The pattern is brought into an associated state by forcing the brain to conceive of it as inside the body.

#8 Smash the mixture into your chest.

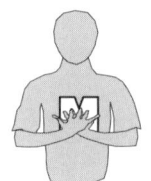

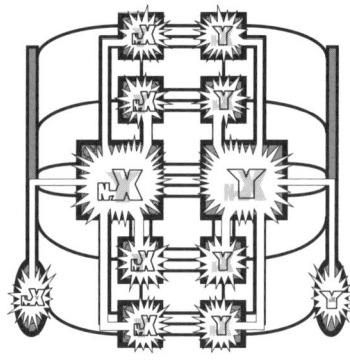

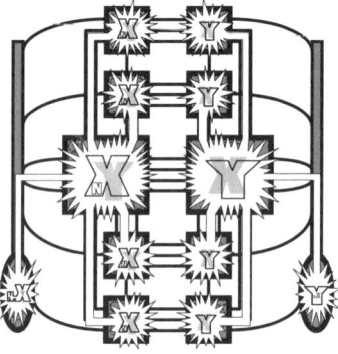

After the brain has boiled with activity for a short time the new pattern is well integrated into the X aggregate.

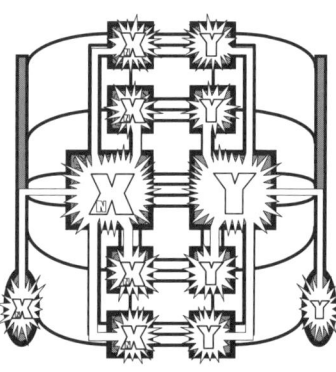

actly like the scenario described here. In truth, patterns are shaped by the perceptions or learnings that we have. Firing up the past, present and future serves not only to excite the areas

Expanded Hammer
Step 9

After installation into the X-aggregate, the new pattern needs to be installed into the Y-aggregate. The steps should be repeated in much the same way, but the new pattern**(N)** starts out in the other hand the second time around.

#9 Repeat steps 1-8, installing the new pattern**(N)** into the other side.

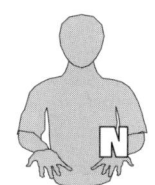

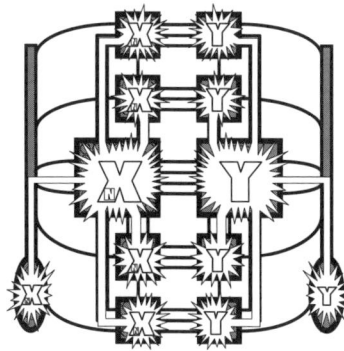

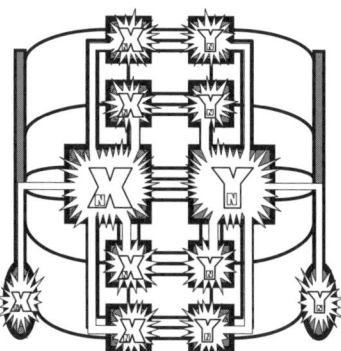

Top left: new pattern has been installed into the X-aggregate.
Top right: new pattern has been installed into the Y-aggregate.
Right: When both sides have recived the new pattern it can be said that the new pattern is a part of the Z-aggregate.

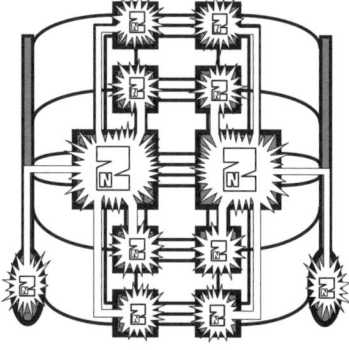

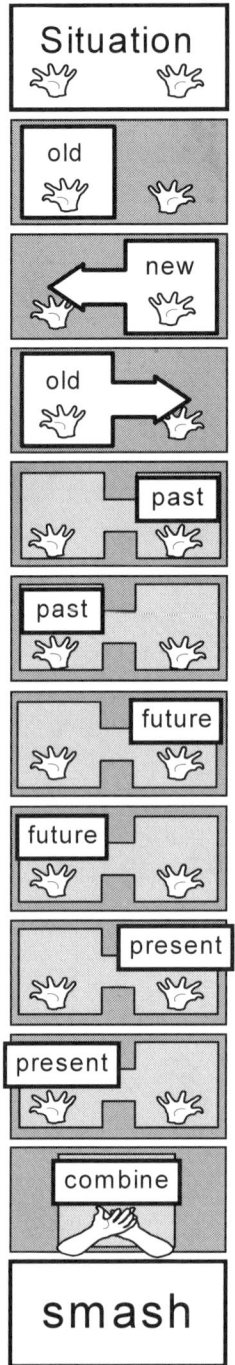

of their involvement, but also to integrate aspects of the new pattern into as much of the brain as possible.

This would seem to be occurring very effectively in actual practice because HAMR produces spectacular results that are nearly imperceptible to the person who is undergoing the change. The change is immediate and thorough with few noticeable side effects.

Other systems of change cause a sensation of strangeness due to the time it takes for the whole brain to integrate new patterns. Perhaps it is similar to the way grief occurs when a person you know and care about dies. Most of the brain does not immediately get used to the idea of the loss that has been suffered, and it feels like you are in another world.

The Hammer. The hammer consists of eight steps that install patterns into *one side of the brain* at a time. Any time a new pattern is installed it should be entered into *both sides of the brain*. Therefore, always preform the hammer once with the new pattern on one hand, then again on the other hand. Failing to do so will create an imbalance that reduces the effectiveness of what you are trying to do.

All of the steps are critical and must be performed completely, or the hammer will not work properly. When dealing with something as powerful as HAMR you cannot afford to be sloppy. You only have one brain, and it has to last your whole life.

This is no time for carelessness.

Omitting steps is asking for trouble. The object is to involve as much cortex as possible without wasting any time. Always be certain to include all of the steps, do them quickly, and do them in order. Your mind is at stake, so make enough effort to get it right.

You do not have to have crystal-clear mental imaging powers; HAMR is not about that. It is not about stressful effort of any kind. It is about taking advantage of superior numerical force and letting your brain do the work.

Fire up the targeted areas of the brain and move on. One important set of areas is the occipital lobes which contain the primary visual cortex. A lot of neurons are taken out of play by closing your eyes, so remember to keep them open throughout all of the steps.

HAMR is designed to be performed with respect to any given situation. It can be exercise, money, relationships, success, or practically any other subject under the sun.

Absolute concentration is not necessary, but it is definitely easier if you can find a nice, quiet place that is relatively free of distractions. What you are trying to achieve is activation of the parts of the brain that are involved with the concept you are modifying at the time.

The hammer-step of putting thoughts in your hands is not meant to be any more elaborate than the familiar concept of "on

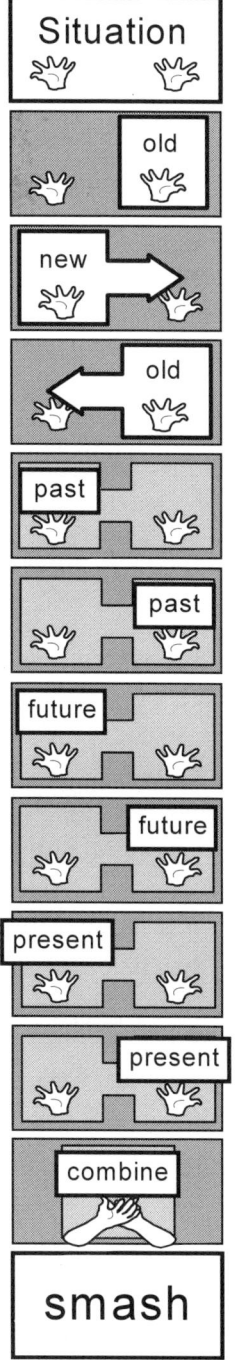

the one hand, I think or feel this way." The hands are neurologically wired up to do this without effort, so there is no need to complicate matters with meditative techniques or deep breathing exercises.

For general purposes the contents called the *new pattern* will be some feeling, wish, or imaginary situation. Many times throughout this book you will see the phrase: "Imagine what it would be like *if*...." In a nice and easy way, you would imagine over in that hand what things would be like if _____ were actually the case. It is critical to imagine what it would really be like because it engages important areas of the brain.

Do not spend large amounts of time pondering early life or its ramifications. The idea is to encourage a normal level of activity in areas of your brain that deal with the past, then go quickly to the next step.

When you get to the last couple of steps, do not worry about whether or not the sides are "ready to go together." They will be cooked into a mutually inclusive pattern and will combine perfectly. Putting the sides together forces the brain to conceive of the new ideas on either side as one integrated concept. Smashing the new conglomerate into your chest forces the brain to conceive of the idea as an associated part of yourself.

A common question is, "Which hand goes on top?" The answer is that it does not matter. Put them whatever way you feel comfortable. It makes absolutely no difference, so do not agonize over your selection.

Now that you have learned *how* to install new patterns of activity on your cerebral hemispheres, you will benefit from knowing *what* patterns to install. From this point *The HAMR Manual* will concern itself with describing what new patterns are effective for improving one's life.

---

[1]R. Bandler and J. Grinder *Frogs into Princes- Neuro Linguistic Programming* (Real People Press 1979)
[2]B. Dilts, T. Hallbom, & S. *Smith Beliefs: Pathways to Health and Wellbeing* (Metamorphous Press 1990)

5

Blitzkrieg

Now that you know *how* to install a new pattern of activity on your neocortex, you need to know *what* pattern to install. Knowing *how* is only a small part of the system whereas knowing *what* is everything.

It is like the old joke about the plumber who shows up at a man's house to fix his pipes. He looks around and scratches his head for a moment, then takes out a small hammer and taps a certain spot on the plumbing. Suddenly everything starts working again, and he hands the guy a bill for $200. The man is incensed and demands to know why tapping a pipe costs so much. The plumber replies, "Look at the bill. It costs $1 for tapping, and $199 for knowing where to tap."

HAMR is exactly the same. Doing the hammer is as easy as tapping on a pipe, but as hard as figuring out exactly where to tap. Without knowledge all the tapping in the world will yield nothing but endless frustration. This chapter will give you the knowledge you need. It provides a systematic approach to fixing your own brain with great ease and effectiveness.

Big Picture. In essence, the goal is to provide your brain with a variety of superior thought patterns. The patterns should enable it to operate more effectively by taking under-used portions of the brain and putting them to work. This is executed by installing thought patterns and attitudes that will get the job done.

The strategy is to take individual situations that exist in life and install aspects of thought patterns that will result in good mental health. Psychology has unearthed a plethora of ideas concerning exactly which aspects of thought are good to have.

Blitzkrieg

Many of the needs we have depend upon certain situations for an opportunity to be fulfilled. Your strategy is to decide which situations you want to master, then make sure that your brain has the full array of positive programming for those situations. There are basically two ways of doing this: search your mind to discover how your brain is mal-programmed then fix it, or simply install everything you need and do not worry about soul-searching. This latter strategy is referred to as **blitzkrieg**.

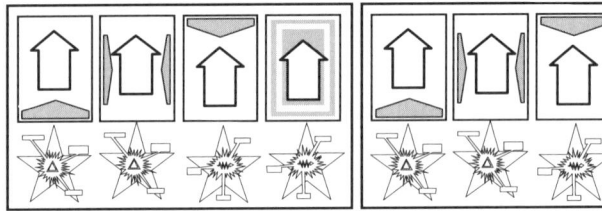

In situations that are of high importance (relationships, money, etc.) it is recommended that you take the blitzkrieg approach. On issues of minor importance or when speed is of the essence, you may want to replace negative patterns with more precision.

The next few diagrams give specific suggestions on what to install while blitzing some of the more critical situations. Going through them is a good way to develop a feel for HAMR and the effects it produces.

**Another very important strategy is to speak with people who are successful at the situation you are working on, then discover and install their beliefs, attitudes, behaviors and right/wrong codes.

Always install positive things and always imagine *what it would be like if* you *already had* the particular thought or attitude. Doing it any other way can cause problems that take up valu-

---

Remember...

The following topical scenarios list basic suggestions for what to install with the hammer (beliefs, attitudes, behaviors, motives and right/wrong codes) to begin improving your life. Each of them must be installed individually (twice, once in each side of the brain) by imagining what life would be like if they were actually true, then doing the hammer.

<u>Very Important:</u>
Always install new patterns by imagining in the new hand what life would be like if (new pattern) was actually the case.

<u>Example:</u> **to install this belief...**

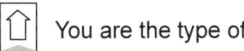 You are the type of person who stays fit

...you would imagine (in the new hand) what it would be like if you actually were the kind of person who stays fit and active.

<u>Example:</u> **to install this behavior...**

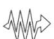 You walk four miles per day

...you would imagine (in the new hand) what it would be like if you actually did walk four miles per day.

<u>Example:</u> **to install this motive...**

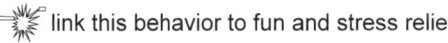 link this behavior to fun and stress relief

...you would imagine (in the new hand) what it would be like if walking four miles per day was really fun and provided powerful stress relief.

The illustration called *Creating Mental Scenarios* (page 70) describes this important concept as well.

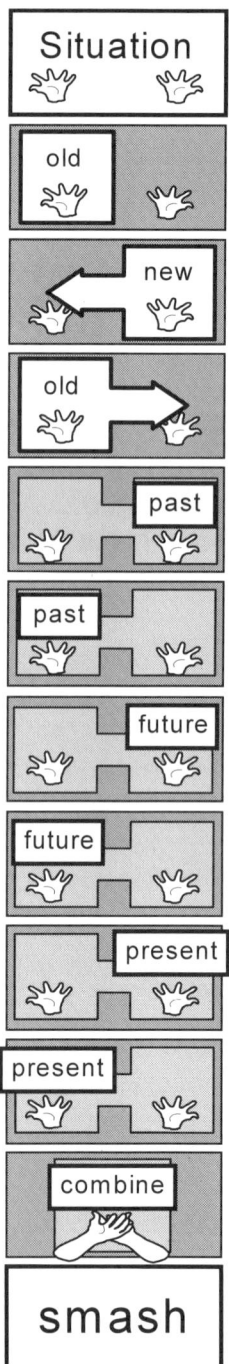

able time to unravel and correct. It may also cause undesirable side effects.

When you imagine what it would be like if things actually *were* better, your brain has the opportunity to evaluate the effectiveness of the new pattern. If your brain determines that the new idea will cause endorphins to be released with a minimal expenditure of energy, it will strengthen the new pattern.

Individual situations that are addressed in this manual are covered in this chapter. They are some of the more widely recognized circumstances in life, and studies show that they are the largest contributors towards happiness.

However, many of the problems that will confront you in life cannot be anticipated in a book that is written by someone else. For this reason it behooves you to have the ability to contrive a strategy for anything that comes your way. At present, many questions remain as to how to apply HAMR to some of the popular demands like weight loss, smoking cessation, etc. Perhaps you will be the one to add such knowledge to the profusion of HAMR's abilities.

Any situation can be improved by adding mental abilities or thought patterns. Adding abilities is the same as adding brain power. You can add abilities or thought patterns, but you can never subtract them (except by surgically removing parts of your brain, which is not recommended).

Adding new patterns that are superior to the old ones is as close as you can get to subtracting, because the brain will abandon the less useful patterns in favor of the better ones. To decide on a course of action that will maximize your potential in a given situation, consider which attributes of thought might make things different.

This chapter tells specifically which patterns have seemed to help in the situations they address. The *blitzkrieg* boxes offer suggestions for producing a well rounded brain. An excellent strategy is to go through the chapter and perform all of the installations in them. Take your time, and give your brain a chance to rest when it feels tired or groggy.

After you have gone through and done all of them, wait a month or so and do it again. Each time you do the hammer unused areas of cortex are activated, and used areas of cortex get to learn the new pattern. When you go all the way through the installations the first time, you are adding more brain power. When you go through all of the installations the second time, you are merging useful patterns into all of the new areas that have been activated.

Big Lincoln Logs First. Take on the problems that bother you most at the time. The bigger they are, the harder they fall. This makes the whole process simple and easy to keep track of. If you do not know where to start, begin with self esteem. Good self esteem will provide the most

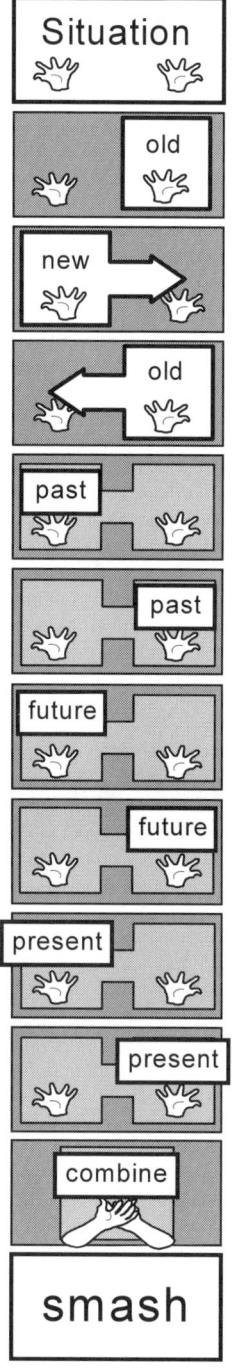

immediate relief available. Over the long term you will need to tackle success, relationships, health, money and religion. If you have any memories that haunt you, HAMR can take the edge off of them by treating the memory as a situation. The entire situational program should be inundated with positive things.

Probably the single most important aspect of a person's thought

Self Esteem

Self esteem can be thought of as self-worth, or how you perceive your degree of importance as a person. Having high self esteem will increase your effectiveness in life and make you a more pleasant person with whom to associate.

Install:

 it is right for you to have high self esteem

 you are a very worthwhile and important person
you are a very mature person

 other people know that you are a very worthwhile, mature and important person

 supernatural beings or forces know that you are a very worthwhile, mature and important person

 things always work out well for you in the end

 you always look at the positive side of things and make the best of every situation

 link this attitude to superiority and satisfaction

 taking care of your own needs first and foremost is the right thing to do

 you always take care of and defend yourself first, and you do not take any flack from anybody

 link this behavior to self respect ,satisfaction and survival

process is the "purpose in life". The chapter called *Success* addresses this issue. No matter how well oiled and smoothly running your brain is, it will go in circles until you aim it at something worthwhile. Self esteem and success should be the first things you take care of. Some people will no doubt ignore this

---

Success

Figure out something you wish you could do that would be worthwhile and would help mankind, mother nature, or both. The occupation you choose will be called (**O**).

Install:

 it is right for you to be in occupation(**O**)

 you are naturally good for occupation(**O**)

 other people know that you are naturally perfect for occupation(**O**)

 supernatural beings or forces are 100% behind you as you do occupation(**O**)

 you will supremely excel in occupation(**O**)

 you always look at the positive side of things and make the best of every situation as you do occupation(**O**)

 link this attitude to superiority and satisfaction

 being successful in occupation(**O**) is the right thing to do

 you are relentless and focused on high achievement in occupation(**O**)

 link this behavior to superiority, self respect, satisfaction and survival

advice and go straight to the box on sex. Be forewarned, how-ever, that you will not be an effective "love machine" with low *self esteem*, so do visit that chapter first.

Use the "Hammerstrips" on the sides of the pages to help you keep the steps in order. Go through this chapter and perform the installations. Each belief, attitude, behavior, motive and right/

Health

Another good place to work hard at being creative and success-ful is health. Attitude has long been recognized for its role in health and well being.

Install:

 it is right for you to have good health

 you are the type of person who is always very healthy

 other people know that you are a very healthy type of person

 supernatural beings or forces know that you are a very healthy type of person

 you will lead a long life and be healthy to the end

 you always try to be health conscious

 link this attitude to self respect, satisfaction, stress relief, better sex, and power

 being healthy is the right thing to do

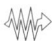 you always exercise, eat right, and have regular medical check-ups

 link this behavior to self respect, satisfaction, stress relief, better sex, and power

wrong-code in the program boxes must be addressed and imagined and hammered individually. Check off each one as you go to assist yourself in staying on track. Install each one twice, once in either side of your brain. After you have finished with all installations, wait a few weeks and do it again.

Money

Fiscal responsibility will be one of the most important skills you ever develop. Use all your creative powers to come up with positive attitudes and behaviors that will do well for you. Pay special attention to right/wrong-coding.

Install:

 it is right for you to be a master of finance

 you are an icon of financial responsibility

 other people know that you are an icon of financial responsibility

 supernatural beings or forces know that you are an icon of financial responsibility

 things will work out well for you in the end money-wise

 you take money seriously, and you are resolved to achieve your financial goals

 link this attitude to food/shelter, safety, wealth, control, power, and superiority

 carefully watching, controlling and growing your money is the right thing to do

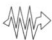 you are the kind of person that does whatever is necessary to achieve financial independence

 link this behavior to food/shelter, safety, wealth, control, power, and superiority

---

Self Esteem. Low self esteem is the most onerous of all obstacles. It saps energy, kills motivation, repels opportunity and eats time. It can also bring about chronic depression. It usually starts when you are young and impressionable, then feeds on any available example of failure as it grows and solidifies. It even causes your body to produce and emit chemical signals

---

Attractiveness

The fact that the elephant man got himself a great looking girlfriend tells us something very important: beauty comes largely from within. If you *feel* good looking you will *be* good looking; and even if that wasn't so, it would still be worth it to install these patterns because it feels great to think you look good, but it feels terrible to think you look bad.

Install:

 for you to feel very attractive is the right thing

 you are a very attractive person

 other people are overwhelmingly attracted and find you irresistible

 supernatural beings or forces conspired to make you a very attractive person just because they like you

 you will be great looking all the way to the end

 you always want to be on your best behavior, and are nice to everyone

 link this attitude to recognition, fun, satisfaction, approval and self respect

 you always take care of yourself and try to look and feel your best

 link this behavior to recognition, fun, satisfaction, approval and self respect

that tell others, "Abuse me, I like it." No thought pattern could possibly be less healthy. Low self esteem is *the enemy.*

Fortunately for us, it is no match for HAMR. To the same degree that low self esteem feels *bad,* high self esteem feels *good.* In fact, it feels great! This simple fact allows the Hebb rule to dominate *low* self esteem *mercilessly.* Having high self

---

Sex

Several thought patterns have demonstrated themselves to have application to the field of sex. Again, talking to people and picking their brains is a great way to get workable ideas.

Install:

 it is right for you to have great sex

 you are a very sexual person

 the types of people that you want sex with are overcome with sexual desire when they are around you

 supernatural beings or forces purposely made you a very sexual person

 you will be sexual all your life, and it will always keep getting better

 you are a person who has just the right amount of control (sexually) over your partner

 link this attitude to superiority, power, fun, excitement, sex, pleasure and stress relief

 taking care of your sexual needs is the right thing to do

 you are a sparkling conversationalist with a propensity to actively get things done (sexually)

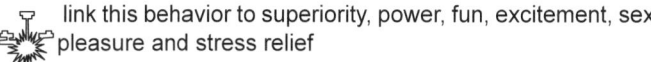 link this behavior to superiority, power, fun, excitement, sex, pleasure and stress relief

esteem not only feels satisfying, it opens up a world of opportunity you never even knew existed. Beliefs are self-fulfilling,
and people pick up on your feelings intuitively.

When you feel good about yourself, other people will also
feel good about you. They will like you, want to be with you
and, want to feel the way you do. You will exude a confidence

Luck

Luck is largely dependent on your state of mind and expectations. To maximize your chances of having good luck and uncan-
nily positive outcomes, install the following thought patterns:

Install:

 it is right for you to have good luck

 you are a very lucky person

 everyone around you is amazed at how good your luck is

 supernatural beings or forces purposely made you a very lucky
person

 you will be lucky all your life, and it will always keep getting
better

 you love having great luck and simply accept its presence as
fact

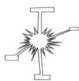 link this attitude to superiority, fun, excitement, power and
safety

 improving your luck is the right thing to do

 you unconsciously do things that result in good luck

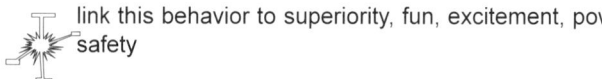 link this behavior to superiority, fun, excitement, power and
safety

that comes from deep within your soul. On such terms life can be very virtuous.

Of all the tools available to you, high self esteem will be the most valuable. That is because barriers will fall away from your path on their own. At last, you will perceive your rightful place in the universe. You deserve a good life, and you must create it for yourself. Fortunately you have what it takes.

Concentration

Good concentration is a necessary ingredient for success in almost any area. To improve yours, perform the following:

Install:

 it is right for you to have powerful concentration

 you are a person who has powerful concentration

 everyone admires your powerful concentration

 supernatural beings or forces purposely gave you powerful concentration

 you will have powerful concentration all your life, and it will always continue to improve

 you enjoy having powerful concentration and know that it will bring you success

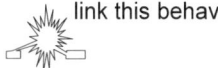 link this behavior to power and control

 having great concentration is right

 you have a powerful ability to focus intensely on your work while completely blocking out distractions

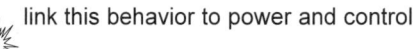 link this behavior to power and control

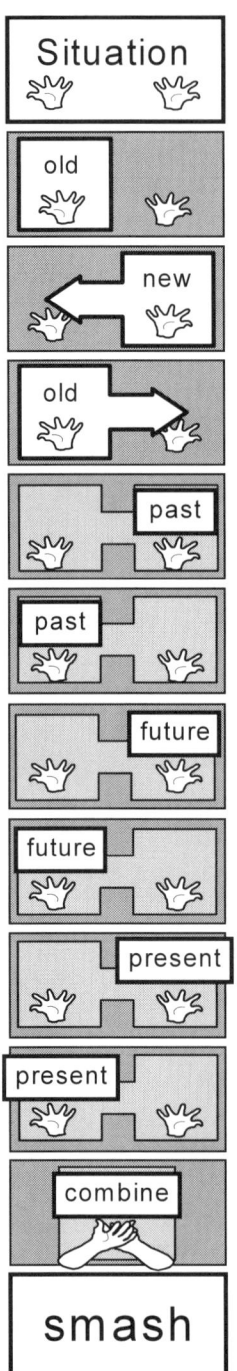

Overview. The idea is to find all negative beliefs about yourself and replace them with positive ones. It may take some time to locate many of them because our brains keep them hidden much of the time (they feel bad). Learn to spot them as you go through life. With the hammer at your constant disposal they can be dispatched when they are discovered any time, any place.

Do not worry about doing everything at once. Get the big problems now and take care of the smaller ones as they become evident. Spend the rest of your life eradicating negative beliefs about yourself and your abilities.

Many contexts and situations exist in your life, and you have beliefs associated with all of them. In addition, your brain and thought patterns are unique; what makes *your* engine run might not do the trick for someone else. It would be impossible to write them all down in one book. Therefore, what you need to do is develop a general "feel" for the HAMR system and tailor it to your own needs. Adding creativity to your array of skills may also be of benefit.

Self Preservation is the first and foremost necessity in the development of good self esteem. A hard cold fact of life is that if you do not put yourself first, you will be of no value to anyone else either. Evolution would not have taken us this far without it. For the good of any species a parent must save itself ahead of saving its off-spring, because without the parent there can be no more propagation or no surviving descendants. Put yourself first so that you can be fit and healthy to care for the ones you love.

Beauty is in the eye of the beholder, and the beholder sees what the beholder wants to see. It is simple: if you feel attractive you will be, and if you feel ugly you will be; therefore, it is better to feel attractive than it is to feel ugly.

Our attitudes, responses, and even the muscles in our faces make it happen. When people feel attractive to other people, they are attractive to other people.

Maturity is a huge factor in the way people treat you. We have all seen people who resort to acting like a child when they do not get their way; observers then feel contempt toward this immature behavior. Psychology refers to this as "age regression" and classifies it as an arrest in development. Whatever it is, it has got to go. Be sure to install maturity from all possible angles.

Success. Doing something worthwhile does not have to be an earth shattering event. All you have to do is contribute in a way that makes your soul come to life. A little bit at a time is enough. No one person is in a position to save the world, but each and every one of us can add to the cumulative effort of making things better.

Many people are looking for that brass

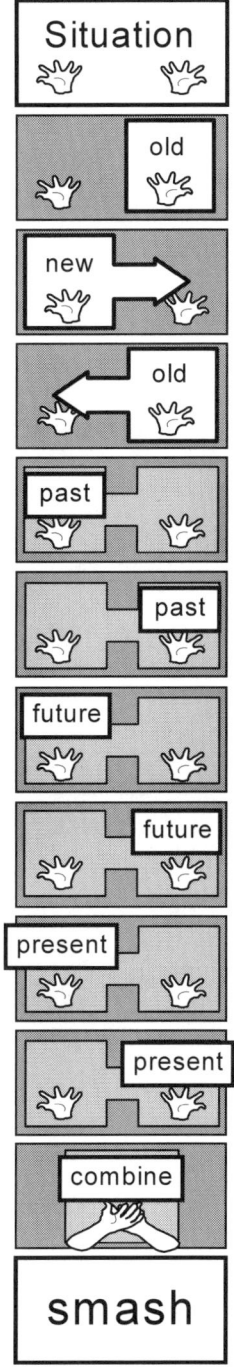

ring of truth that will show them their secret purpose in life.
They think that one and only one activity will satisfy their search
for meaning. This is an error, and it brings about a tremendous
waste of valuable time and talent.

Nobody knows where their journey will take them until they
arrive somewhere. The road we travel leads into the future, and

---

Optimism

Having an all around positive attitude has many benefits. Your
chances of success, health and general sense of well being will
be enhanced by the following patterns:

Install:

 it is right for you to be optimistic

 you are a very optimistic person

 people admire your optimism and wish they could be like you

 supernatural beings or forces purposely made you a very optimistic person

 you will be optimistic all your life, and it will always keep getting better

 you feel that you might as well make the best of things with the
time you have

 link this attitude to happiness, approval and recognition

 maintaining your optimism is the right thing to do

 you always try to do the right thing and make the best of any
situation

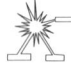 link this attitude to happiness, approval and recognition

there are no maps to follow. Forget about the magical elixir of perfect attainment. Your job is to get up and try to lend a hand in any way that you can. The human race is about to be in a world of trouble, and it will take effort from all of us to avert disaster.

It may be that you dream of doing something in particular that you feel will assist. If that is so then by all means go for it

---

Creativity

Enhanced creativity is always useful. Do not hesitate to install this entire battery of patterns to any situation in which success is vital:

Install:

 it is right for you to be naturally creative

 you are a naturally creative person

 everyone knows that you are naturally very creative

 supernatural beings or forces purposely made you a very creative person

 you will be creative all your life, and it will always keep getting better

 you have a philosophy of doing things creatively

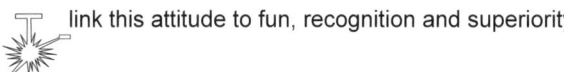 link this attitude to fun, recognition and superiority

 being creative is the right thing to do

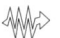 you always try to find creative ways of doing things

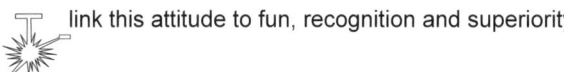 link this attitude to fun, recognition and superiority

with all your heart and soul. If you do not have such an idea, welcome to the club. Most people are in the same boat in that respect. However, if you can get rolling with the idea of making a positive contribution of some sort, the universe will smile upon you, and you will find purpose. A worthwhile human being can ask for no more and settle for no less.

Exercise

Install the following mental patterns to increase the likelihood of exercise. Always start slowly and work up, and always stick to something that you can enjoy for a long time.

Install:

 it is right for you to exercise regularly

 you are a very active person

 everyone knows that you are a very active person who exercises regularly

 supernatural beings or forces purposely made you a very active person

 you will be a very active person all your life

 your attitude is that good health and well-being depends on staying active

 link this attitude to survival, power, fun and stress relief

 exercise is the right thing to do

 you make a point of staying active and fit

 link this attitude to survival, power, fun and stress relief

The strategy for attaining success is to install the necessary drive and or motivation to get things going as well as a set of beliefs that will allow your brain to kick into full gear. The motivation will no doubt be disguised as a wish for some "unattainable" goal.

As mentioned, if you already have something worthwhile that you would like to do, by all means wire it up and go. Bear in

Spirituality

To increase your spirituality, install the following thought patterns. Tailor it to your own particular religious preference.

Install:

 it is right for you to be spiritual

 you are a very spiritual person

 everyone knows that you are a very spiritual person

 supernatural beings or forces purposely made you a very spiritual person

 you will be spiritual all your life, and it will always keep getting deeper

 you always keep an open mind and stay in touch with your spirituality

 link this attitude to happiness

 taking care of your spiritual needs is the right thing to do

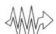 you keep in touch with your spiritual self

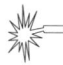 link this behavior to happiness

mind, however, that most of life's highest achievers started out wanting to do something other than what they actually did.

A few suggestions may be in order to get you moving: half of the earth's oxygen is produced by tiny patches of rain forest that are quickly being chopped into toothpicks and cigar boxes. Population explosion is placing mankind at increasing risk for

---

Public Speaking

From time to time, many of us are faced with the task of addressing a group of people. The more confidence you can have in such a situation, the better it will go. The following thought patterns may offer some assistance:

<u>Install:</u>

 it is right for you to speak in front of a group

 you are very talented at speaking to groups

 the people in the audience are very interested in what you are saying, and they think you are great

 supernatural beings or forces purposely made you so good in front of groups

 you will be talented at speaking to groups all your life, and it will always keep getting better

 you are always up for public speaking because you love doing it

 link this attitude to superiority, power, recognition, control, fun and excitement

 speaking to groups of people seems very *right* for you to do

 you are a sparkling conversationalist and are always ready to jump up and speak to a group

 link this behavior to superiority, power, recognition, control, fun and excitement

widespread epidemics, hunger, and plagues. Every minute we lose several species of plant and animal forever. Many of the medicines and cures for diseases we discover are in these plants and animals. The human race is cutting short its chance for survival with chain saws and smokestacks. We need to take a wide variety of action in this regard.

Assertiveness

Some people have trouble standing up for themselves, and some have trouble keeping their aggression in check. The following patterns should improve either situation:

Install:

 it is right for you to assert yourself with just the right amount of force

 you are an assertive person who is also in perfect control

 everyone knows that you are reserved normally, but will stand up for yourself without hesitation

 supernatural beings or forces purposely made you an assertive yet perfectly controlled person

 you will maintain exactly the correct amount of assertiveness forever

 your philosophy is to always be nice to others, yet assertive enough to protect your own interests

 link this attitude to control, survival and self respect

 asserting yourself enough to protect your own interests is the right thing to do

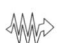 you are always nice to others, yet assertive enough when it comes to protecting your own interests

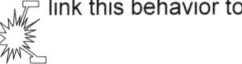 link this behavior to control, survival and self respec

Pollution is getting worse, animal species are dying off, and the hole in our ozone layer is getting bigger. We need chemists, doctors, environmentalists, biologists, *honest* politicians, and a host of other scientific dedicates. In short, we need people who do not like what is happening to the earth and are willing to do whatever it takes to rectify the situation.

Stress

A certain amount of stress is good, but too much at a time for long periods is detrimental. Installing the following thought patterns, can help you to keep it under control:

Install:

 it is right for you to keep stress under control

 you are the kind of person who keeps stress under control

 everyone knows you are the kind of person who keeps stress under control

 supernatural beings or forces gave you the ability to keep stress under control

 you will have the ability to minimize stress all your life, and it will keep getting better

 your philosophy is to minimize stress

 link this attitude to survival, stress relief and control

 taking care of yourself and not stressing out is the right thing to do

 you to minimize stress by stopping and concentrating on relaxing when you need to

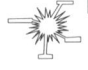 link this behavior to survival, stress relief and control

Be forewarned: after your brain has been amended to accomplish such tasks, you will likely be subjected to a wide range of emotional turbulence. This upheaval will take the form of primal dissatisfaction, sadness, and regret at the amount of time wasted so far. Do yourself a favor and go easy on the self criti-

---

Strong Finishes

Highly successful people have a common behavioral-thread that runs through all of them: they finish what they start. They go into a task with the intention of completing it, and they pour it on at the end. If you want to improve your follow-through, install the following patterns:

Install:

 it is right for you to always finish what you start

 you are the type of person who finishes strongly

 people around you admire how you always come up with a powerful finish

 supernatural beings or forces purposely made you a very strong finisher

 you will finish strong all your life, and it will always keep getting more powerful

 your attitude is that if you are going to start something you may as well be prepared to finish it

 link this attitude to superiority, power, self respect and wealth

 being a powerful and unstoppable force that finishes strongly feels very right for you

 towards the end of a project, you are powerhouse that can taste success and pours on the effort the end

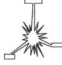 link this attitude to superiority, power, self respect and wealth

---

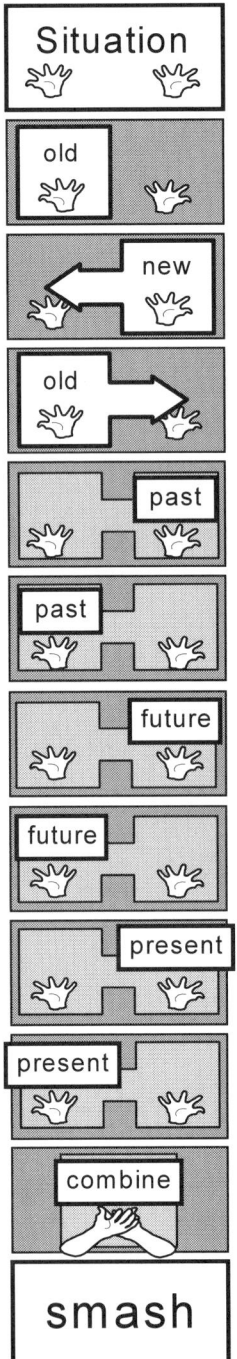

cism. Recall that you have indeed done the best you could with what was available. After all, HAMR has not been there for you until now.

Health. It has long been known that a positive attitude can improve your health. The placebo effect is a well-documented phenomenon. Some of what this chapter does is to induce placebo, and some of it is designed to encourage healthy living.

It goes without saying that if you are sick and dying, there is not much you can do for anyone else. Good quality of life will require good health. It would be tragic to work hard for many years, finally accomplishing your dreams, only to die as a result of your own bad habits. Good health will also give you the energy to accomplish great things. Doing something worthwhile for the universe will require an amount of effort that is over and above the norm. Bear in mind also that with the advent of HAMR the competition is about to become *much* stiffer.

You must charge forward with abandon or be left eating the dust of those who do. Making it big on planet earth will also demand longevity and good staying power. It takes a long time and a lot of dedication to accomplish most worthwhile things, especially in science. You will need to live your life with the idea of making it endure forever. The last one standing wins.

The underlying mechanism that ties attitude to health remain largely unknown.

There have been correlations drawn between moderated expression of anger and blood pressure, but the evidence is still sketchy. Much remains to be discovered in this area, so for now HAMR will concentrate on installing positive attitudes and healthy habits.

Mating. How others perceive us is strongly affected by our own ideas of how they see us. Mating is not based on looks, charm, talent, or even money. It is mainly dependent upon confidence, and confidence is on HAMR's turf.

The first order of business is the development of good self esteem. If you have not completed everything in that section, go back and finish it now. Self esteem is critical to the development of good poise, and you will need the full range of emotional response to come across evenly.

People are attracted by confidence and repelled by desperation. Therefore, the idea is to wire up your brain to expect a positive outcome in social situations. Since self confidence feels good and gets wonderful results, the Hebb rule kicks in nice and hard. Other people will suddenly seem to change their attitudes, but the root cause is in your own thoughts and actions.

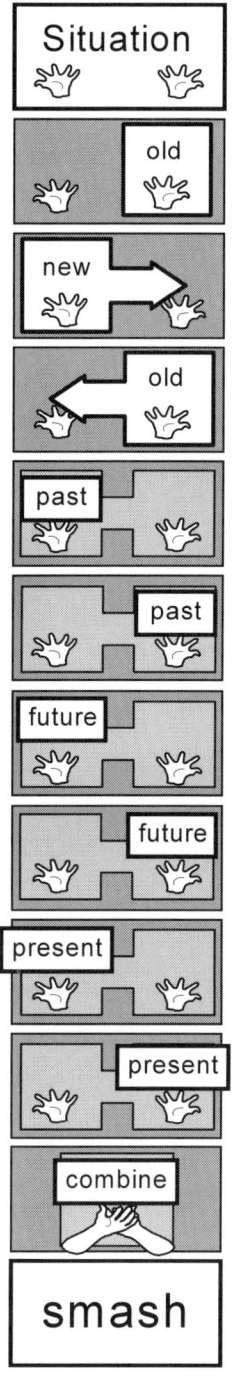

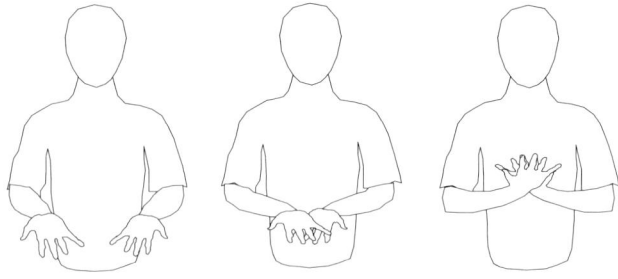

6

Epilogue

Many anthropologists today believe that the human race has absolutely no chance of survival. They say that our unrelenting spree of self destructive behavior has already taken us past the point of no return. We have annihilated millions of species of plant and animal, destroyed countless acres of oxygen-producing rain forest, and polluted the lakes, streams, and oceans of our planet to the point that much of it will no longer sustain life.

Many countries are so permeated with land mines that they are uninhabitable. The population is exploding, nuclear bombs are increasingly at risk of falling into the wrong hands, and diseases are mutating into deadlier forms.

Some people think that striking out into space will provide an answer, but living in space is not an option for a species that cannot even live in the environment in which it evolved. Eventually there will come a time when something has to give, and that time is coming faster than people realize.

The question is: what are *you* going to do about it? In your hands, you now have the ability to master your own brain. You can do whatever you want to do, and you can compete with the big boys. It is the opinion of this author that we can turn the situation around and make our race a competitor in the universe; however, it can only happen if we start immediately, and aggressively pursue it. We need to stay alive, and to do that we will need to save what is left of our mother, the earth. We need scientists, environmentalists, and business people who care about what is going to happen.

This book was written with the intention of providing *you* with the ability to master *your own* mind. The system is very easy to use, and its power outstrips anything that has been devised so far. It represents a new direction for modern psychology. It does not matter if you believe it will work; it only matters if you *do* it.

The HAMR system is still in its infancy, and the situations that are addressed in this edition are only the beginning. However, it remains a very real possibility that the hammer is capable of eradicating a sizable portion of what we presently term *mental illness*. It is hoped that this book will stimulate the interest of research-minded individuals.

The theory behind HAMR is base upon neurology. The description that is offered herein is designed to strike a balance somewhere between accuracy and simplicity. It is not meant to be taken as absolutely correct, but there may be some truth to it. Any theory must be polished and improved by the sands of time, and HAMR is no exception.

Your brain is made up of billions of neurons, each one communicating with thousands of others. They communicate by either inhibition or facilitation, and they stimulate each other to activity. The result of this stimulation is chaotic in nature, but from the chaos is born order and meaning. To produce this meaning the whole brain works together. Many discreet areas make contributions toward the overall process.

The object of HAMR is to tease out more useful patterns, then bring the level of chaotic activity to a high enough level that the newer and better patterns become solid. If the patterns are useful to the brain as a whole, we assume that the Hebb rule will apply, and the brain will grow new connections to facilitate the new patterns. Thus the term: "rewiring the brain."

The Hebb rule will only apply if a reward is garnished as a result of the new patterns of activity; therefore, we always attempt to install patterns that are positive and useful. The issue then becomes how to decipher which patterns satisfy these requirements.

While we refer to this process as *rewiring the brain*, it should be noted that the situation is actually a bit more complicated than that. New patterns can be established, and new branches can be grown over time to strengthen the patterns, but old branches cannot be removed readily. An analogy would be pathways through a dense forest. New paths can and will be established through usage if they are useful and provide a more direct route to some reward. But the old ones that are well trodden will remain for a long time, and if they are needed can easily be reused.

The human brain can be functionally divided into two hemispheres and four lobes. The frontal lobes seem to be specialized for differing emotions, aspects of situations, and approach-withdrawal type behaviors. The left anterior frontal lobe is responsible for approach-related behavior, and it uses emotions such as interest, anger, and desire to facilitate its action. The right anterior frontal lobe is responsible for withdrawal-type behavior, and it uses emotions such as fear, distress, and disgust to facilitate its action. All successful interaction with the environment must consist of some combination of the two.

Both cerebral hemispheres are capable of maintaining their own separate beliefs. Each hemisphere is specialized for differing tasks and will only attempt a given task if it possesses a reasonable expectation of success. For this reason it is standard operating procedure to install positive beliefs in both sides of your brain each and every time.

Installing patterns is accomplished by doing the hammer. The hammer is a sequence of steps that is designed to merge new patterns into the whole brain at once. It is achieved by firing up parts of the brain that process the past, present, and future at the same time.

The recommended approach is to go through the chapter called Blitzkrieg and install all of the patterns that have little symbols next to them. Put a check by each one as you go along in order to keep track of what you have done so far. After finishing all of them, wait a month or so and do it again.

By the time you get through all of that, you should have a pretty good idea of how HAMR works and what its effects are. Coming up with your own custom-made hammers will be easy, and you may even want to apply your new found skills to helping other people.

HAMR is just getting started, and people like you are in control of its future. Innovations will be made as time goes by, and future editions of the HAMR Manual will recognize the people who come up with them and outline their applications.

Do not hesitate to send correspondence in this respect to Billings Worldwide Brain. Your efforts are appreciated. Best wishes to you in your quest to improve yourself and the world.

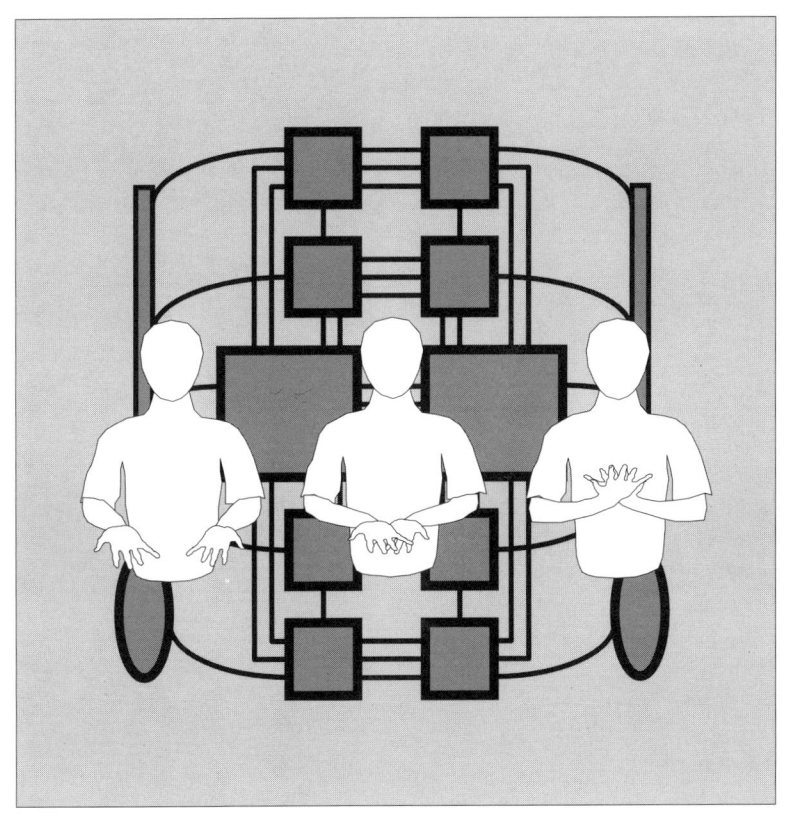

Index

U

unconscious mind   39

V

visualization   18, 20

W

will   39, 81
willpower   28
wish   57

Table of Illustrations

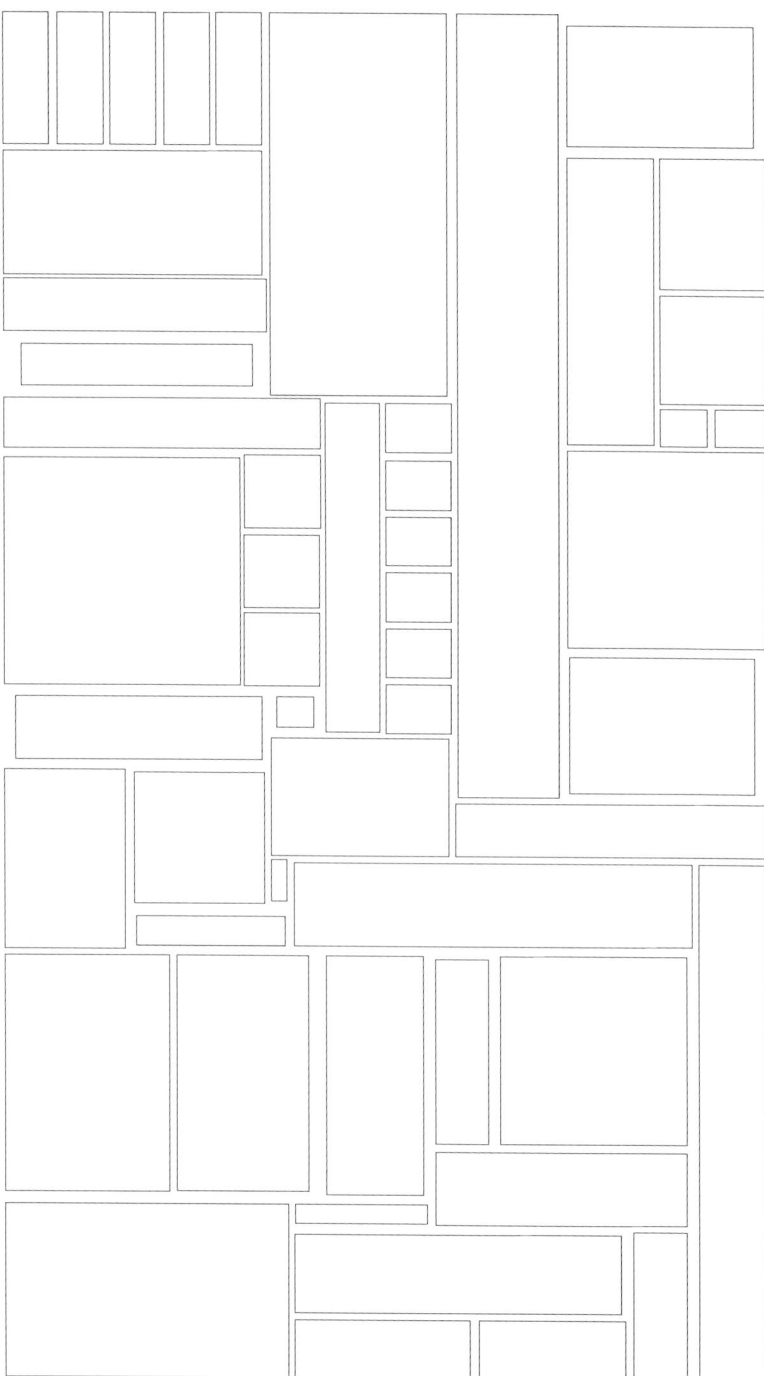

Order Form

Please send [____] **copies of**

The HAMR Manual

I understand that I may return The HAMR Manual at any time, for any reason, for a full refund.

The HAMR Manual: **$19.95 X** [____] **=** [_____]

Texas residents add: **6.25%**   **X .625**

Shipping & Handling: **$2.00 1st book**
                   $.75 each additional book

Total Enclosed $[_____]

Send check or money order payable to:

Billings Worldwide Brain
P.O. Box 701
Addison, Texas 75001

Name: _____

Address: _____

City, State, ZIP: _____

*Note: you do not need to send this form to order a book. Simply send your check or money order for the correct amount along with all of the information requested below.

Order Form

Please send ☐ copies of

The HAMR Manual

I understand that I may return The HAMR Manual at any time, for any reason, for a full refund.

The HAMR Manual: $19.95 X ☐ = ☐

Texas residents add: **6.25%**   **X   .625**

Shipping & Handling: **$2.00 1st book**
                         $.75 each additional book

Total Enclosed $

Send check or money order payable to:

Billings Worldwide Brain
P.O. Box 701
Addison, Texas 75001

Name: _____

Address: _____

City, State, ZIP: _____

About the NCEO

The National Center for Employee Ownership (NCEO) is widely considered to be the leading authority on employee ownership in the U.S. and the world. Established in 1981 as a nonprofit information and membership organization, it now has thousands of members, including companies, professionals, unions, government officials, academics, and interested individuals. It is funded entirely through the work it does.

The NCEO's mission is to provide the most objective, reliable information possible about employee ownership at the most affordable price possible. As part of the NCEO's commitment to providing objective information, it does not lobby or provide ongoing consulting services. The NCEO publishes a variety of materials on employee ownership and participation; holds dozens of seminars, Webinars, and conferences on employee ownership annually; and offers online courses. The NCEO's work also includes extensive contacts with the media.

Membership Benefits

NCEO members receive the following benefits:

- The members-only newsletter *Employee Ownership Report*.
- Access to the members-only area of the NCEO's Web site.
- Free access to live Webinars.
- Discounts on books and other NCEO products and services.
- The right to contact the NCEO for answers to questions.

An introductory one-year membership costs $90 for U.S. residents. To join or order publications, telephone us at 510-208-1300 or visit our Web site at www.nceo.org.